Edible and Medicinal
Mushrooms
of New England and Eastern Canada

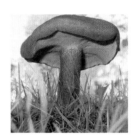

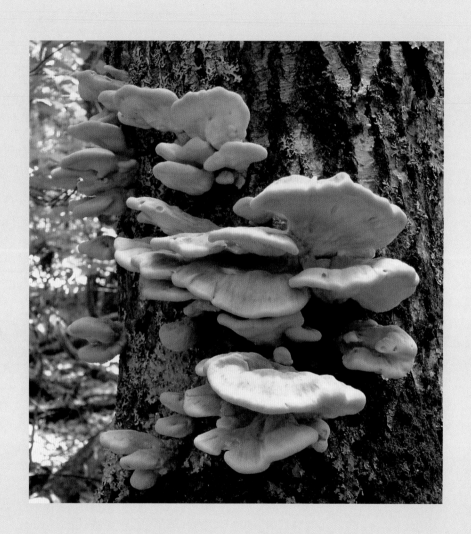

Edible and Medicinal

Mushrooms

of New England and Eastern Canada

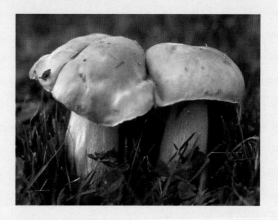

David L. Spahr

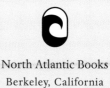

North Atlantic Books
Berkeley, California

Published by
North Atlantic Books
P.O. Box 12327
Berkeley, California 94712

Except where noted, all photos are by the author.
Cover and book design by Brad Greene
Printed in the United States of America

Edible and Medicinal Mushrooms of New England and Eastern Canada is sponsored by the Society for the Study of Native Arts and Sciences, a nonprofit educational corporation whose goals are to develop an educational and cross-cultural perspective linking various scientific, social, and artistic fields; to nurture a holistic view of arts, sciences, humanities, and healing; and to publish and distribute literature on the relationship of mind, body, and nature.

North Atlantic Books' publications are available through most bookstores. For further information, visit our Web site at www.northatlanticbooks.com or call 800-733-3000.

Library of Congress Cataloging-in-Publication Data

Spahr, David L., 1950–
  Edible and medicinal mushrooms of New England and Eastern Canada
/ David L. Spahr.
    p. cm.
  Includes bibliographical references and index.
  ISBN 978-1-55643-795-3 (trade pbk.)
  1. Mushrooms—New England 2. Mushrooms—Canada. 3. Cookery (Mushrooms) I. Title.
  TX558.M9S63 2009
  641.6'58—dc22

                                                    2009001698

    1 2 3 4 5 6 7 8 9 SHERIDAN 14 13 12 11 10 09

Dedicated to my mother, Mary L. Spahr—who recognized my interest and gave me my first mushroom book—and to all of those who share my love of nature and the beauty it offers.

Disclaimer

There is risk to ingesting wild mushrooms; illness and even death can occur. Some mushrooms that are safe for most people may make some people ill. The author makes no warranties as to the safety of consuming wild mushrooms and accepts no liability or responsibility for any consequences resulting from the use of, or reliance upon, the information contained herein, nor for any health problems, consequences, or symptoms that may arise from contact with or the ingestion of mushrooms and other fungi herein described. Any person who ingests mushrooms or any other potentially dangerous fungi does so at his or her own risk. Be sure to learn rules for collecting and refer to additional books. When in doubt, throw it out(side)!

Contents

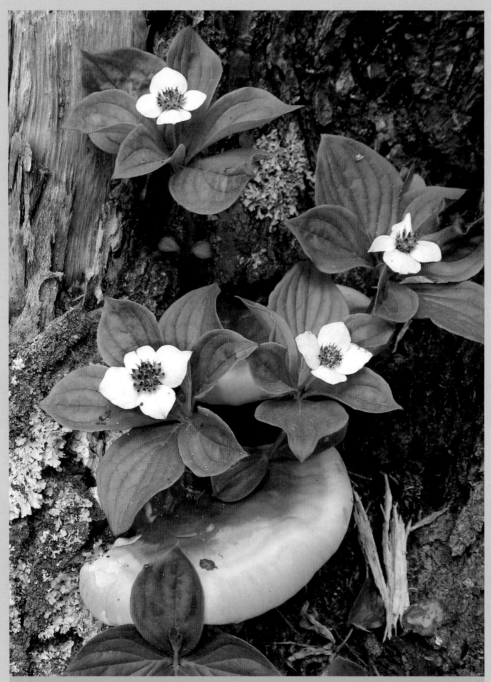

Hemlock Reishi *(Ganoderma tsugae)* and Bunchberry *(Cornus Canadensis).*

Preface

Follow this guide for finding, collecting, identifying, and preparing the more safe and common edible and medicinal mushroom species of New England and Eastern Canada.

I live in the town of Washington, Maine, located in Knox County, midway between central and midcoast Maine. I am known by some as the Mushroom Maineiac. Nearly all of the species in this book are gathered and photographed within thirty-five miles of my residence. I created and photographed all content unless otherwise noted. Additionally, I have personally ingested almost all of the edible species I describe.

There is risk in consuming wild mushrooms; this is a learning process that can take a lifetime. One should not go right out and pick! First, read a comprehensive field guide, find an experienced teacher or a club, learn the rules for collecting, and be very careful.

It is extremely important for you to realize that mushrooms listed as edible in some field guides may not be edible in *your* area. For example, the Lilac-brown Bolete *(Tylopilus eximius)* is usually listed as edible; however, in Maine, there have been many poisonings from this species. Do not eat it. Another example to be avoided is Angel Wings *(Pleurocybella porrigens),* a thin and white Oyster-like mushroom found growing on conifers. There have also been some reports of poisoning recently although most field guides list Angel Wings as edible—avoid them.

This guide offers you inside information on finding mushrooms. During the past decade, when I wanted to be able to locate new species, I would often ask other mushroom hunters, brokers, and others how I would find mushrooms, such as Matsutake or Black Trumpets. I most often received general or somewhat sketchy descriptions of how to locate them. Many are protective of their knowledge and "their" mushrooms. Field guides tend to give a mycological general description of the ecology, such as "several to gregarious under hardwoods and sometimes conifers in the eastern United States from July to September." I do not find a description like this particularly helpful and avoid such dry, general descriptions.

This guide provides useful ideas for cooking mushrooms. Many people look at the different types of mushrooms and are not sure how to prepare them. Mushrooms, like vegetables, have widely varying flavors, textures, and colors. Water absorption among the distinct species can range from "soaks like a sponge" to "floats like a cork." Most mushrooms only respond well to certain cooking techniques. Generally, it is not wise to mix wild mushrooms with White Button / Cremini / Portobello Mushrooms (all *Agaricus bisporus*) from your supermarket unless you want your wild mushrooms to taste like the strong-flavored *Agaricus bisporus*. Porcini and Maitake may maintain their character but the Chanterelle flavor is easily lost. Many wild mushrooms—like fine wines—are just too rare, subtle, or distinctive in flavor to be mixed or combined in certain ways. It makes as much sense as using Château Lafite Rothschild to make holiday punch!

In the Northeast we are blessed with many of the very best medicinal mushrooms available. The medicinal species treated here all grow on wood. This guide will increase awareness of these species and their unique healing components. Information has been gleaned from respected resources, such as PubMed from the National Institute of Health Library, the

American Cancer Society, Sloan-Kettering Cancer Center, and other scientific sources. Presently, however, there are ambitious assertions about mushrooms that may not have adequate scientific backing being generated by some who are selling mushroom products on the Internet.

Mushrooms may be used for dyeing fabrics and paper. Anne Williams of Stonington, Maine, generously shares the discoveries of her many years of research in dyeing wool with mushrooms. She also makes unique mushroom yarn, which you can purchase.

This is not a traditional field guide. It does not identify every mushroom found in the Northeast. That is not in keeping with the purpose of this guide. The general field guides do that exceptionally well. This guide is also not about hallucinogenic mushrooms. Do not try to pick hallucinogenic mushrooms! Little brown mushrooms can be very difficult for even mycologists to identify. For instance, eating a *Galerina* by mistake could result in death!

This book is about the easy-to-find, relatively safe, edible, and medicinal mushrooms found in New England and Eastern Canada. Most of the species included are found in many parts of the world. However, I have omitted some mushrooms with questionable relatives, or that are hard to find, flavorless, or of questionable edibility. *Leccinum* species (Scaber Stalks) and Slippery Jack *(Suillus luteus)* are not covered although they are listed as nonpoisonous in most books. These two examples fail on two counts: they do not agree with some people and they have marginal culinary value.

I have collected and consumed wild mushrooms since 1973. Good information about edible mushrooms was hard to find in the 1970s, so I was fortunate not to poison myself. That said,

I was actually quite careful, eating only large Puffballs and Fairy Ring Mushrooms at first. I endeavored to add one or two species a year to the mushrooms I was eating. It was not until 1981 when the *National Audubon Society Field Guide to North American Mushrooms* by Gary H. Lincoff was published that I started to become serious about collecting. I liked Lincoff's use of common names and tried to learn the accompanying Latin names of the mushrooms I cared about. I have referred to that book countless times, studying it from cover to cover.

I have the heart of a hunter, farmer, and cook more than the heart of a scientist. I have a forager's mentality. I have loved everything outdoors since I was old enough to go outside. We had farm property and lived right next to the woods so I spent a lot of time there. Close encounters with wild and domestic animals, plants, and trees were daily occurrences.

My mother taught me many things about plants, including flowers as well as edible and poisonous plants. I learned about purslane, pigweed, herbs, and many other wild plants being edible. She showed me some deadly nightshade and warned me not to touch it because it was poisonous. Her identification was incorrect—the deadly nightshade was actually pokeweed, which is also poisonous so the advice was still good. When I was a child, she warned me away from "toadstools." She did not know about mushrooms.

So many other things outside interested me that this was not important. I dug a lot of holes and rolled over lots of rotten logs. I played in the woods every day. I picked black raspberries with the girl next door throughout the summer. Few things in the world were more interesting to me than salamanders, frogs, and turtles. I had many temporary pets.

Our mother also taught all of us how to cook at a very young age. My youngest brother, Andy, became a chef. I worked in restaurants for many years in a variety of capacities including as a cook. I have loved cooking all of my life.

My dad was a mechanical engineer by day and a farmer when he came home from work. He had studied both engineering and agriculture in college. We raised chickens, ducks, pigs, and other animals for our sustenance. He also maintained a large vegetable garden, which he taught me how to plant from age four. I loved making squash hills and dropping the seeds down the rows. We ate some of the wild rabbits that were eating our vegetables. He took me fishing for brook trout at the ponds at the bottom of the hill many times. We ate a lot of trout when I was growing up. I never realized as a child how necessary all these things were to our existence. My parents did not have much money to support their modest farmhouse but we certainly ate well.

Part of the property was leased to a local beekeeper, Charlie Oikle. I loved to see Charlie coming. I would run up the hill and from a distance watch him maintain his hives. He always taught me some facts about bees when I visited and always had a free pint of honey to offer.

Later we moved to an architect-designed Victorian home with a barn, circular driveway, formal gardens, stone walls, hedges, bushes, orchards, a large vegetable garden, and so many types of trees. It was a wonderful place that my parents purchased for a bargain price. We had many heirloom apple trees, pears, peaches, a walnut tree, mulberry tree, grape arbors, and other types of trees and bushes. The local extension service was very interested in our property because of the number of different scarce trees, bushes, and plants we had. We worked a lot on our property as kids to maintain it because we could not afford to hire people. It took seven hours just to mow the lawn. I dreaded picking up apples except when we were pressing cider.

My brother John became a beekeeper when he was about ten years old. He made money from selling the honey and we always had all the honey we wanted. Andy had chickens so there were more than enough fresh eggs to sell and eat. I raised racing and fancy pigeons. It was an idyllic existence. My brothers and I fished a lot and were always bringing home different kinds of wild fish to eat. Andy, who eventually became a chef, used to jig for frogs and cook frogs' legs for us.

When other kids were going to YMCA summer camp, I went to nature training school, where I learned more about water life, birds, insects, forest trees, ecology, and other subjects. I loved science in school and began my college career majoring in biology (not where I ended up). This love of nature and the outdoors has persisted throughout my life. It was only natural that I would eventually want to know about the Fairy Ring Mushrooms near one of our apple trees.

When I first began collecting edible mushrooms, the Internet did not exist and there were no online mushroom groups. I did not know anyone else who did this and was not aware of any clubs so the learning process was slow. I heard stories about mushroom collectors, but they were not mycologists. I heard a story about an Italian man who collected certain mushrooms in the woods, another about a man who went to great trouble to harvest a mushroom from the crotch of an elm tree, and yet another about a woman who collected Fairy Ring Mushrooms. I learned somewhere that Puffballs were edible if they were white inside.

I had no technique other than to try to learn about mushrooms I spotted by chance or by just walking in the woods. I was learning to be a photographer, and mushrooms were a good subject to photograph. In the beginning, my photographic skills were not of the level necessary to get many clear, well-composed photographs.

Over the years as my knowledge increased, my enthusiasm gained momentum. I did meet a few knowledgeable people along the way. I owe a debt of gratitude to Mike Dubois of Mexico, Maine, who taught me things about edible mushrooms and got me thinking about stump culture back in the 1980s and '90s. Mike was an herbalist known as the Maine Ginseng Man. We talked a lot about mushrooms and woodland farming, and I have acted on some of the ideas we discussed. Unfortunately Mike passed away at a young age.

I only recently joined the Maine Mycological Association (MMA) and attended a few of their organized group forays. MMA has many knowledgeable mushroom experts and fanciers to learn from. It was an honor to learn from Dr. Samuel Ristich, the founder of MMA and one of the original mushroom gurus. I cannot say I learned enough from Dr. Ristich, but his knowledge, attitude, and enthusiasm was truly inspiring.

I certainly respect peer-reviewed scientific methods of inquiry and understand how that differs from anecdotal evidence. I do use a microscope occasionally for learning and identification. I culture spores and grow spawn but mostly for the purpose of growing mushrooms around my house and woodlot. Rather than having a lot of logs or a growing room, I am attempting to inoculate fresh stumps and induce growth of local wild (and other) species around my property, using slurries, transplantation, plug spawn, and other strategies. I am a compulsive experimenter. I envision my woodlot and surrounding property as a mushroom and wild plant wonderland in a few years. Some strategies are my own ideas and as yet of unproven worth. Because I have a lot of ideas, I am seeing which ones will "stick to the wall." I have been doing this since the early 1990s.

Mushroom Collecting Basics

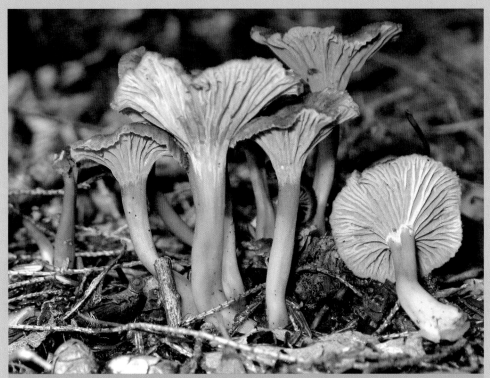

Winter Chanterelle *(Craterellus tubaeformis)*.

Chapter One

Collecting Edible and Medicinal Mushrooms

What Is a Mushroom?

Mushrooms are organisms that belong to the kingdom of fungi. The fungi kingdom encompasses more than 100,000 species, including molds, yeasts, and mushrooms, with many more species still to be discovered and classified.

Technically a mushroom is not a plant. Mushrooms are static and have cell walls. The cell walls of fungi are composed of chitin rather than cellulose. Instead than carrying out photosynthesis, fungi must absorb food from their surroundings by releasing digestive enzymes to decompose both living and dead organic matter in the environment.

Mushrooms are called *macrofungi*. They are the fruiting body of a perennial underground network called *mycelium,* the main part of the organism. Harvesting a mushroom is much like picking a fruit from a tree. Mushrooms will continue to grow each year for as long as the growing environment will support the mycelium. The mycelium is critical to the environment in decomposing the molecules of trees, plants, and animals. Many are *saprobic,* deriving their energy from dead organic material. More than ninety percent of all living plants form symbiotic relationships with fungi. The mycelium absorbs carbohydrates from the plant while delivering water and minerals to the plant.

Rules for Collecting

Be sure to purchase a authoritative field guide, such as *National Audubon Society Field Guide to North American Mushrooms*. Refer to more than one book.

1. Make a positive identification using more than one source wherever possible. Do not eat mushrooms with any features that contradict the description. Contact a mushroom expert or club if you are not sure. If you are still unsure, heed the advice: "When in doubt, throw it out!"

2. Only pick specimens with opened caps because mushrooms can easily be misidentified in the button stage.

3. Keep your known edibles separate from unknown specimens. Any unknown mushroom is possibly dangerous.

4. Take notes on all of the important aspects of the environment, including types of trees, plants, other fungi, soil, forest or land characteristics, and any other unusual aspects of the location. It is best to write it down and keep your notes with your specimens.

5. Use every aspect of the mushroom's physical structure for identification, including a spore print. Spore prints should be made on black or white paper or glass.

6. Be able to distinguish a mushroom species from its close relatives and unrelated look-alikes.

7. Learn what deadly species look like and the symptoms of poisoning.

8. Avoid picking any little brown mushrooms and difficult to

identify or poisonous species, such genera as *Amanita, Galerina, Entoloma,* and *Cortinarius.* Beginners should also avoid mushrooms from the *Lepiota, Lactarius,* and *Russula* genera. Learn the basic characteristics of these genera so that you can avoid them.

9. Never eat any bulbous-based gilled mushroom growing from a sac or cup. Those are likely to be *Amanitas*—many species of which are deadly.

10. Avoid Boletes with red or orange pores that stain blue. Mushrooms that stain blue when cut or bruised should always raise a caution flag, although a few can be eaten. For beginners, mushrooms that stain black are best avoided, too.

11. For beginners, it is safer to start by collecting mushrooms with pores, teeth, and ridges rather than gilled mushrooms.

12. Avoid polluted, treated, or sprayed areas. Weed-less lawns should be avoided. Fruit tree orchards should be avoided unless you know for sure they have not been sprayed. Pesticide residues can remain in the soil for many years—possibly decades. Lead arsenate remains in the soil even longer than the DDT that succeeded it.

13. Do not pick next to busy paved roadways. There could still be lead in the soil from leaded gasoline we used to burn and cadmium from rubber-tire dust. On busy roadways, pollution spreads from cars in a way similar to the dust cloud behind a cattle stampede.

14. Realize that there are no simple rules of thumb about edibility, such as "if it stains a silver spoon . . ." or other generalizations.

15. Do not damage the environment. Avoid picking or knocking over mushrooms that you do not intend to keep. Fill any holes in the dirt or duff so the underlying mycelium

does not dry out or become damaged. It is best not to use a rake for finding Matsutake. A good mushroom hunter leaves few traces behind.

16. Always cook your mushrooms thoroughly. There are bacteria in the outdoors and you could become ill from something entirely unrelated to the mushroom.

17. Only consume fresh specimens. Older specimens may be spoiled.

18. Chew them well and eat only a small quantity.

19. Try one new species at a time, eating only a small amount at first and retaining a sample of the new species in case of poisoning or allergic reaction. Just as some people cannot eat nuts, strawberries, shellfish, or other foods, allergic responses to some mushrooms are certainly possible.

20. When fall rolls around and the hunting seasons begin, wear hunter orange in the woods at all times.

As with all rules and descriptions there are always exceptions. Size of mushrooms in particular can be quite variable. I have been puzzled on quite a number of occasions by mushrooms that were much larger than descriptions indicate. Every once in a while you will find twelve-inch or larger Boletes, Horse Mushrooms, Oyster Mushrooms, or others. I have learned that a ten-inch Blewit is definitely possible. Because 2006 was a wet year, Chanterelles commonly had four- to six-inch caps. Size can be confusing, so understand that size can be much greater than field guide parameters suggest. Even very experienced collectors can sometimes have trouble with identification. Mushrooms can have very different looks at different stages. Factors, like sun and moisture, can greatly affect the look of an easy-to-identify mushroom.

Collecting Tips

Know your trees. This is imperative. Many good edible mushrooms are *mycorrhizal.* They develop a symbiotic relationship (friendly exchange) with trees or other plants. Fungal mycelium, intimately joined to the roots of a tree, receives carbohydrates and other nutrition from tree while delivering minerals and water to the tree. The tree often receives a significant amount of its water intake by delivery from the mycelial network extending far beyond the reach of the root system. Both organisms benefit. Mycorrhizal fungi cannot live without the tree, and the tree will struggle without fungi. Fungi can also be *saprobes,* which consume dead organic material in the ground or the dead or dying tissue of living trees. Saprobes tend to prefer certain hosts. Similarly, parasitic fungi that destroy and consume living tissue tend to be particular about which trees, plants, fungi, or animals they infect.

In Maine, recognizing oak and hemlock is an absolute requirement. You need to know about many other tree and plant species as well. *National Audubon Society Regional Guide to New England* is a good reference. Learn to spot the species of trees from a distance.

Eastern Hemlock associates with dozens of species of mushrooms, such as King Boletes, Chanterelles, Matsutake, Aborted Entoloma and other tasty Boletes are found on the ground. Mature trees will usually be more productive. Hemlock Reishi *(Ganoderma tsugae)* and other shelf mushrooms fruit on dead wood.

Oak supports many species, including Maitake, King Boletes, Chanterelles, Black Trumpets, Chicken of the Woods, Blewits,

Honey Mushrooms, and Oyster Mushrooms. For Maitake and many others, look for large, mature trees with possibly some dead wood in the tree. Oak stands with young and middle-aged trees are usually not as productive and are best avoided. I often find Maitake growing near oaks that are infected with Honey Mushrooms.

Under **Eastern White Pine**, look for Chanterelles, Painted Suillus, Chicken Fat Mushrooms, other species of *Suillus*, *Boletus pinicola/pinophilus* (a type of King Bolete), and a few others.

White, yellow, and other birches can harbor Chaga and other Polypores on the wood as well as Chanterelles, Hedgehogs, Boletes, and other species on the ground. Mature, scarred, or dying trees usually produce more.

Beech woods are a prime area for Black Trumpets. Chanterelles, Oyster Mushrooms, and Hedgehogs are occasionally associated with beeches.

Maple is a common host for Oyster Mushrooms in fall and early winter *(Pleurotus ostreatus)*. In particular, sugar maple is the most likely host. Again, look for mature, dying, and dead trees. I have found *Boletus bicolor, Craterellus ignicolor,* and *Craterellus tubaeformis* near maples. That said, most activity around maple is likely to be on the wood rather than on the ground with such species as *Pleurotus ostreatus* (Oyster Mushroom), *Pleurotus dryinus, Polyporus squamosus* (Dryad's Saddle), *Panellis serotinus* (Late Fall Oyster) *Volvariella bombycina, Ganoderma applanatum* (Artist's Conk), and *Climacodon septentrionale* (Northern Tooth) occurring fairly commonly on the wood.

Poplar/Aspen is a common host for Oysters Mushrooms *(Pleurotus populinus)* in May and June. Turkey Tails are often found on poplar. Many other types of fungi also find poplar to be a friendly place to grow.

Balsam Fir (the Christmas tree), very common in Maine, often hosts good stands of Chanterelles or Boletes beneath it.

Spruce varieties support a wide variety of mushrooms. Blue spruce, although not native to this area, is fairly common in planted stands and lawns. Blue spruce supports King Boletes, Chanterelles, and many other species. Black spruce tends to grow around swamps, streams, and sphagnum bogs. Red and white spruce tend toward rockier soil and hillsides. Positive identification of spruce varieties can be a challenge. All support mushrooms.

Mature, dying, or dead trees should always receive extra attention. Maitake, Oyster Mushrooms, Chicken of the Woods, Reishi, and Turkey Tails are found almost exclusively on this type of substrate (growing medium). Look for trees that woodpeckers have been working on. Large, mature oaks and sugar maples with dead branches always have excellent potential. Sometimes spotting trees that support mushrooms is easier in the winter. You can always be looking! Chaga and Artist's Conk can be found year round and will sport easy-to-spot "snow hats" after a storm. Oyster Mushrooms are occasionally found in winter during extended warm periods.

Cuttings where wood was harvested a few years earlier have many stumps where various types of mushrooms may grow. This is especially true for selectively cut woodlots that still offer some shade. Wood-harvesting equipment, like skidders and harvesters, often cause scarring on remaining living trees where various fungi may get a start. I have birches on my property that have Chaga growing from these types of scars.

Look for mixed woods. Mixed hardwoods and conifers provide numerous habitats. Many varieties of mushrooms may be found there. Whereas, planted tree stands with just one variety of tree, such as eastern white pine or red pine, are often unproductive. People have advised me to look for Matsutake under red pine. I have found red pine stands, however, to be particularly barren except for False Morels.

Pastures and other areas with very rich soil from manure are places where Meadow Mushrooms, Horse Mushrooms, Puffballs, and other good coprophilic (dung-loving) mushrooms can often be found. Be on the lookout from July through November at these locations.

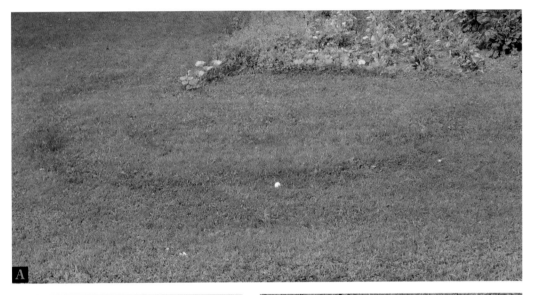

🍄 **Figure A:** This shows a ring of greener, taller grass where a fairy ring of *Agaricus campestris* is starting to grow. Mushrooms tend to grow just to the outside of the dark ring. The substrate inside the ring is likely used up so the underground mycelium moves outward forming a ring.
🍄 **Figure B:** This patch may form a ring next year.

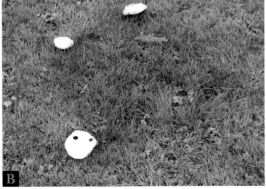

Look for dark green patches or rings in lawns or pastures. Dark green areas of grass are often locations where Meadow Mushrooms, Horse Mushrooms, and Puffballs will soon appear. However, you must find out whether herbicides have been used on the lawn. One clue is to look for weeds—a weedy lawn is far less likely to have been treated.

Search edges of parks, cemeteries, and trails, and along dirt roads. Wherever grass clippings and leaf compost are deposited are good places to find Blewits in the late fall. Cemeteries are always worth a look if they are old, not treated with herbicides, and mowed only a few times a year. There is apparently far less herbicide usage in Maine than in Massachusetts and points south. Weeds are also a useful indicator for mushrooms. Woodland trail edges and edges of shaded country dirt roads are often productive and obvious. My theory is that the compacted soil of trails and roads may prevent the mycelium from spreading inducing it to fruit.

Embankments that are shaded by trees, such as oaks or hemlocks, most of the day are fine places to look. Trails and back roads where the banks are covered with a thick bed of sphagnum type mosses beneath trees are an excellent bet, too. The south side of a road or trail is likely to be shadier and mossier. You might notice that on an east to west stretch of tree-lined road that the south side is mossy and the north side is grassy or quite barren.

Mosses of the brushier type, like the various species of sphagnum moss, often have mushrooms growing on or near them. Mosses are a strong indicator when found on an embankment.

Search near streams, lakes, ponds, bogs, and coastal areas. These are microclimates where fog; wet ground; humidity; and other factors, such as plentiful dead wood and leaves, tend to produce mushrooms and other fungi. Coastal areas usually have a different distribution of tree species with oak being more plentiful.

Explore washes. Washes are intermittent streams on hills, on small mountains, and in valleys where water rushes through during spring runoff and heavy rainstorms. Sometimes the water will actually create natural dams of dead trees or branches that fall, are washed down the hill, and become lodged sideways behind living trees. A stone wall or a large rock can also create a dam. Mushrooms, such as Black Trumpets and Chanterelles, tend to proliferate in washes below these dams. Washes can often be followed long distances with phenomenal results (bring your GPS). Shady is better. Once I understood that washes were prime locations, Black Trumpets seemed to be everywhere.

Smell the air. Sometimes you can actually smell mushrooms. A large stand of Black Trumpets has such a strong smell that you may be able to pick up from a distance. Mushroom-filled woods often have an earthy smell.

Useful Equipment

Mushroom collecting can be done inexpensively with minimal equipment. You may already have most of the necessary items. However, there are some things you may want or need should you become more serious about collecting. Below is a list of some items a well-prepared collector may want and still be able to travel light.

Vest or backpack: A vest, such as one for a fisherman or photographer, is excellent for carrying the items listed below. A good backpack with compartments is also useful but somewhat less convenient.

Field guide: A reliable reference, such as the *National Audubon Society Field Guide to North American Mushrooms* by Gary H. Lincoff, is highly recommended. Books by Roger Phillips and Miller & Miller are also reliable references but are not pocketable.

Notebook and pen: Taking notes about the location and habitat of your specimens is very useful, and a GPS text entry is even better.

Magnifying glass: Some sort of magnifying lens is practically a requirement. I carry a 10x folding loupe in my pocket at all times. But this need not be expensive; for instance, even a household magnifier would work.

Basket, mesh bag, or other bags: Carry at least one medium- to large-sized basket. There are many inexpensive choices. For example, collapsible nylon shopping baskets with a light aluminum frame and drawstring top work well and are fairly easy to carry. Paper grocery bags also work and are easy to carry and free. Plastic is fine as long as you transfer your specimens to another more suitable container, like a basket, soon afterward. Leaving mushrooms in plastic for too long on a warm or hot day causes them to sweat and become soft and slimy. A mesh bag is easy to carry, breathes, and may distribute spores. The mesh can rough up delicate species, though. What you choose as a container also depends on what you hope to collect. A plastic bag is excellent for Chaga. But for extra large species, like a giant-sized Maitake or Chicken of the Woods, I use a large, shallow plastic tub, which is sometimes even too small. You may spot mushrooms when you least expect to and do not have all your equipment handy. For these times, I try to keep a basket, bags, and some equipment in my vehicle. When I hunt it is often a process of driving to a place and getting out to harvest for just a few minutes and moving on. A hot car can be a serious problem with a covered container or one that has poor aeration so quick collections and transfers to other containers are often best.

Wax or brown paper bags: Keeping the mushroom species you are not sure about separate is imperative. Unidentified species that are potentially poisonous should not touch your known edibles. Therefore, segregate unknown species in brown paper lunch bags or wax paper bags, usually available in supermarkets.

Mushroom knife: To avoid getting unnecessary dirt in your collection basket, use a knife to cut your finds. A bit expensive and sometimes hard item to find locally, a mushroom knife usually has a brush on one end for brushing off your finds and a small curved blade on the other. A pruning knife or other sharp knife, such as a Swiss army knife, is fine. If you choose a conventional knife, you may also want to bring a mushroom brush or small paintbrush. Knives tend to dull quickly when coming in contact with the ground, and sharpening them in the field is often impractical. Once knives have become dull, they tend to pull the whole stem out of the ground. In some cases it is best to pull up the entire mushroom rather than cut it. You may need the entire stem to study or use the stem butts for propagation. The mycelia at the bottom of the stem will often regenerate if the environment is friendly. It is unacceptable to cut a Matsutake for the Japanese market.—only untrimmed specimens are marketable.

Utility scissors: An inexpensive pair can be very useful while collecting. For instance, I like using scissors to harvest Chanterelles, which tend to pull out of the ground when using a dull knife.

Garden trowel: If transplantation interests you or you want some mycelium for further study, a trowel is a useful tool.

Hatchet: For harvesting Chaga *(Inonotus obliquus)* and other hard shelf mushrooms, a small hatchet is usually necessary.

GPS with WAAS and maps: An optional item, GPS offers a sense of security about not becoming lost in the woods if you want to follow the mushrooms wherever you find them. WAAS units are accurate within three meters. Built-in maps make navigating and locating your best finds easy by saving track logs, waypoints, and other valuable markers. I start by marking the location of my vehicle before entering the woods. I bought a Magellan Explorist 200 for a bit more than $100. Maps and memory are self-contained. More expensive GPS units often have removable memory cards or attach to your computer's USB port for information exchange.

Bug repellant and attire: Failing to wear bug repellant and a *hat* can ruin your day. I usually spray the repellant on my hat and sometimes my socks and clothing rather than my skin. I use Deep Woods Off! *Gloves* can be necessary when the Chanterelles are in or around the poison ivy. Digging in the dirt often brings you in contact with poison ivy roots. Wearing gloves also makes handling possibly poisonous species safer. *Shoes* or *boots* made for hiking should be worn for protection and comfort. In the places I frequent in Maine, I often need waterproof boots. Tucking your pants into *tall socks* is smart during black fly and no-see-um season and also helps to avoid deer ticks. Main carriers of Lyme disease and other diseases, deer ticks are one of the biggest dangers mushroom collectors face. When leaving the woods, I always check for ticks and often find them. A deer tick will often crawl around on your skin for twelve to twenty-four hours before deciding where to bite.

Whistle: Should you become lost or injured, a whistle is a handy thing to have to help someone find you. A cell phone is even better.

Walking stick: Use it to push bushes, ferns, or other plants aside while you hunt as well as for photographing mushrooms. A photographer's monopod can easily double as a solid, light, collapsible walking stick.

Photographing Mushrooms

Recent advances in digital camera technology have changed the face of digital photography. I have used digital cameras starting with the first Sony Mavica for quick online auction listings and Web-page photos. I was not impressed with the resolution (1.3 megapixels) for "real" pictures, though—until now. Small point-and-shoot cameras can have so many advanced features that carrying around suitcases of equipment is no longer necessary. Most of the photographs in this book were taken with a point-and-shoot digital camera. Be aware, though, that a small camera can be hard to operate if you have large hands and that it has been my experience that a small camera can easily slip out of a pocket.

A digital camera that can capture 5 megapixels of information or more is recommended if you want quality pictures of your mushrooms and still be able to travel light. Cameras that can capture from 6 to 12 megapixel images are quite common. Better digital cameras are equipped with macro (close-up) functions and various exposure modes. Most will have auto, program, aperture priority, shutter priority, manual, and even video modes. I think using a camera with aperture priority and manual mode is a must.

A single lens reflex camera (SLR) is not a requirement for taking good pictures of your finds. For some photographers, SLRs really are necessary for sports action, telephoto, or technical photography; but for most people, an advanced-feature point-and-shoot camera will certainly meet your needs. SLRs do offer fine optics and the versatility of interchangeable lenses, but they are heavy, awkward, and require carrying a lot of extra equipment to utilize their slight advantage. The good macro capabilities and many exposure functions of the more advanced point-and-shoot cameras make carrying a lot of equipment unnecessary. They are pocketable. This is quite helpful for a mushroom hunter who may end up with bags or baskets of fruit bodies to carry out of the woods. I now carry a camera virtually everywhere I go and get so many more pictures of all aspects of my life than I ever did when I was using 35mm SLRs.

The woods can be quite dark and program or auto mode will give a correct exposure but often not enough depth of field (focus). Aperture priority mode is an essential feature to have to get better depth of focus because the aperture remains at your selected setting while the camera adjusts the shutter speed accordingly. You can also use manual mode to achieve similar or better results if you can outthink your camera. I really like the manual function on my Canon Powershot A630 because rather than having a needle or LED indicator, the image on the viewing screen gets lighter or darker as you adjust the shutter speed so what you see is what you get. The closer you get, the more necessary it is to "stop down." Comparable lenses by different manufacturers are usually very similar in sharpness. Sharpness varies much more by f-stop (aperture) than by camera brand. Most lenses perform with optimal sharpness and contrast in the f-4.5 to f-11 range. However, f-4.5 and 5.6 may not yield suitable depth of focus if your camera is really close to the subject. My Canon Powershot A630 only stops down to f-8. Other cameras using f-16, f-22, or f-32 will certainly give greater depth of focus but will require much longer exposure times and less sharpness due to diffraction. Bracketing your exposures may be a good idea in some cases. Software often cannot restore burned out highlights or underexposed shadow areas. A digital camera's CCD can only cover a few f-stops of dynamic range within the frame. It is best to expose your image to maintain highlight detail. Shadow noise is muddiness and poor detail in the darker image areas caused by lightening an image with photo-editing software. Shadow noise is easier to deal with than a burned out highlight, though. Conventional film still has a considerable edge in interpreting the darks and lights at the extreme ends as well as much greater resolution. A color slide can be made into an 80MB file.

It should be noted that the on camera flash will often help but can be hard to use at very close distance often yielding burned-out highlights and high-key, somewhat unnatural-looking colors. When correctly used, though, the flash can help to enhance colors. Your camera's built in flash is likely to be too weak at distances greater than six to ten feet. If you are going to use flash, it is often better to stand some distance from your subject and zoom in just a bit, but more than five feet

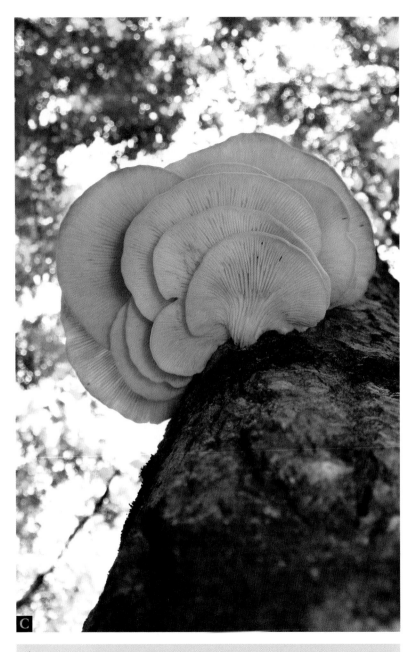

🐾 **Figure C:** This is an example of using flash in a backlit situation. I exposed this photograph of *Pleurotus populinus* with normal exposure set to minus 1/3 f-stop and flash set to minus 2 f-stops.

away is likely to be too far. Note that the greater the lens' focal length, the less depth of focus so it is best not to get carried away with zooming in. Greater focal length (zooming in) also requires greater steadiness. If I need to get close, I often set my flash to minus 2 stops and expose normally or at minus 1/3 f-stop using flash to because shooting pictures in this way requires slower shutter speeds. Using a white card as a reflector can be useful in some cases. A piece of cardboard covered with aluminum foil works well, too. I use flash almost all the time. What I try to take is an image that looks like flash was not used; well lit, but without the dark background, harsh shadows, and high-key subject area so often seen in photographs using a high-power flash. The size and shape of your subject often dictates the distancing and camera position. A large Maitake allows more options than a tiny mushroom.

There are many bright-light situations when you should use flash. If your subject is strongly backlit, using your flash is necessary for high resolution of the main subject. For example, looking up a tree at a large flush of Oyster Mushrooms where the sky is the background, the hymenia (undersides) of the mushrooms would be too much in shadow for good detail. There could be greater than 5 stops of variation of light intensity in this situation so you would use flash to fill the shadows, thereby lighting the underside of the mushrooms. Photographing a scene like this both with and without flash is usually a wise idea. When using the flash to fill dark areas, you may want to back your flash power down a couple of stops. Take a lot of pictures. Experiment with your settings. Use your image view setting to be sure you have taken the picture you want before you leave the scene.

Camera and Film

Sometimes, your best pictures will be taken using available light. Many digital cameras now have image stabilization, which can help greatly by often allowing you two more f-stops or shutter speeds. You may be able to get a fairly sharp photograph hand-held at one-fifteenth of a second if you are very, very steady. The other solution is stabilization using a tripod, monopod, or beanbag. Often, you can place your camera right on the ground for stabilization too. You will need to become accustomed to crawling or lying on the ground. I occasionally use the top of my shoe or my knee for greater steadiness. With a digital camera, you should not hesitate to take a lot of pictures. Memory cards are inexpensive and can often hold hundreds of pictures. Review and delete your "less than excellent" pictures as you go. Because image view mode allows you to zoom in to see how much sharpness there is in critical subject areas, you know before you have left the scene if you have the pictures you want. Sometimes I may take five hundred pictures in a day, deleting more than three hundred in the field. The ability to review and delete or edit your photographs immediately is one way that digital has 35mm beat. Five hundred photographs taken with Fujichrome ISO 100 would cost almost as much as the camera. The three hundred film images are money down the drain.

When making pictures with 35mm film, one generally tries for precise framing at exposure. As a student and professional photographer, I was very tuned-in to doing this. Careful in-camera cropping is important when using a 35mm SLR and most always requires quite a bit of extra time. Previsualization of exposure is very important. Because wasting film is expensive, bracketing of exposures often necessary. Digital photographs are very easy to crop on a computer so tight, precise cropping is less necessary. You can leave a bit more space around your subject, which allows you to shoot from a greater distance, resulting in greater depth of focus and apparent sharpness. You can often use just a small portion of a digital photograph that did not have enough depth of focus in all areas of the frame.

Often those photographers who stick with 35mm photography feel that conventional films give a more accurate and "real" interpretation of the scene. In terms of contrast and resolution, you do get excellent results with 35mm photography. Anyone who has loaded two cameras with different films, such as Fujichrome and Kodachrome, will find that each film yields very different results of the same subject with the same exposure. Films can have very different palettes. I highlight these two film examples because the differences in interpretation are quite dramatic. Try to remember, films are simply different paint boxes. Ektachrome yields colors more similar to Fujichrome. A digital camera that could be set to a Fujichrome or Kodachrome color palette would be very cool. Slide films are by far the best choice for 35mm photography both from the contrast and resolution standpoint as well as for publishing and storage. In the recent past, editors and graphic designers often wanted transparencies (slides). That is changing. Today, they usually prefer digital files. Slides are easier and better to scan than negative film and can be scanned as ultrahigh-resolution TIFF files and easily converted to other formats.

Digital photography is closing the gap. High-resolution photographs can be made with newer cameras. Especially useful are those that can make RAW files, which are minimally processed images that are easily edited, printed, or converted to an RGB format, such as JPG or TIFF. Usually only more expensive digital SLR cameras capture images in the RAW file format, but that situation is changing. When taking digital photographs with a higher-resolution camera, composing the image tightly is far less necessary because cropping is exceptionally easy with a computer and a photo-editing program. Dodging, burning, and color adjustment is also far easier when editing on a computer. Any adjustments made can easily be undone before saving the finished image. For 35mm photographers, though, a change of mindset is required when changing to the digital format.

I have a Canon Powershot A630, 8 megapixel, camera that I like quite well. It is pocketable (big pocket) but is not too small. The screen flips out and swivels to many different positions, making photographing next to the ground, overhead, or photographing yourself much easier. Because of its versatility, size, and weight, I take mine most places; and as a result, I have never taken so many pictures spontaneously.

If you do not mind hauling a lot of equipment, there are many digital and 35mm SLR's to choose from, which is always a good solution for high-quality pictures. But you are no longer traveling light. I personally like and recommend Fujichrome ISO 100 film for vivid color.

For Canon Powershot cameras, you can get CHDK firmware files, which enhance the firmware functions of your present camera. Small files are installed in the root directory of your camera's memory card and can be enabled when you power on your camera. Your camera's original firmware is not altered. CHDK is always evolving and firmware versions are available for many functions. CHDK can override and expand your shutter speed selections, f-stop choices, ISO, and have depth of field and color map graphics. Most versions allow you to shoot RAW files. There are special builds for fast motion, stereoscopic, and other specialized applications. They can be downloaded free from the Internet. For more information, go to http://chdk.wikia.com/.

Mini-tripod

A mini-tripod, or a regular tripod, is almost mandatory for photographing in aperture priority mode with no flash if the lighting conditions are challenging. The pocket tripods with the flexible legs seem a bit flimsy, but they work better than you might expect. An exceptionally innovative yet inexpensive flexible tripod called a Gorillapod is well suited for mushroom photography. I have the smaller version that is quite small, but I really like it. It sits really low and it grabs on to all sorts of inanimate objects. The tripod block is exceptionally small so I can leave it mounted to my camera and not even notice it. This allows me to slide my camera quickly onto the head of the tripod and lock it on with a definitive snap. There is also a version available for the larger SLR cameras. Using your self-timer with your tripod will help you get sharper pictures.

Monopod

A monopod is also very useful, especially one that collapses to be fairly short. In addition to using it on the ground, I sometimes use it with the base lodged behind my belt buckle for sharper handheld pictures taken from a standing position. Use the monopod as a walking stick and to push aside bushes, ferns, or other plants as you hunt. I have even used mine to knock high-growing Oyster Mushrooms from trees.

Beanbag

This photographer's secret is such a handy item to have and so easy to carry. Often you need to photograph a specimen on or very near the ground. Using a beanbag for support offers you great steadiness and positioning, which can yield very sharp pictures. In many situations a beanbag is better than a tripod because it is less affected by wind or vibration and you can more easily get a very low angle of view. Once you settle the camera into the correct position, using the self-timer for "hands off" exposure will render a sharper picture. You may want an additional beanbag for supporting a slave flash. Make your own simple, easy beanbag by pouring uncooked beans or rice into a sock and tying it closed.

Auxiliary Flash with Slave and Other Accessories

A small flash with slave unit for wireless synchronization can be quite useful for adding extra light for exposure and some side or backlight for a more natural look. The problem you can run into is that most digital cameras have a preflash for red-eye that can fire the slave prematurely, creating the light burst too soon. You can shut off the red-eye flash setting on most cameras. It is best to leave it shut off for photographing mushrooms when using auxiliary flash. You may find that you can resurrect an older flash and slave that way. An even more sophisticated solution for flat lighting is the Sunpak FP-38 E-Flash, On-camera Flat-Light Kit with Mounting Bracket and Built in Slave. Your mini-tripod or a beanbag can come in handy for supporting the auxiliary flash. You will need to experiment with different setups to get the kind of look you want.

Through the years I have learned that it is wise to be prepared and have extra supplies available while in the field. So I always carry extra memory cards and batteries.

Mushrooms with Gills, Ridges, or Teeth

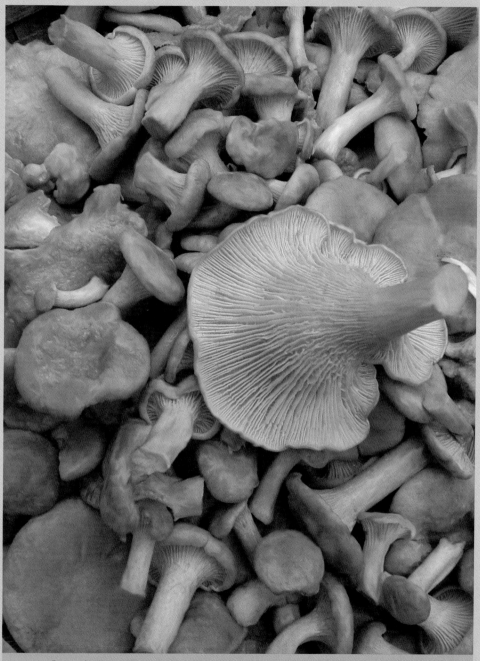

One afternoon's bounty, showing normal size and shape variations of the Chanterelle.

Chapter Two

Chanterelle

(Cantharellus cibarius)

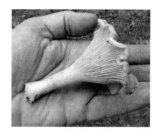

This Chanterelle is a large beauty of normal color.

T he Chanterelle is found and enjoyed by people all over the world. In Europe it has many names, such as *Pfifferling* in Germany, *Girolle* in France, and *Gallinacci* in Italy. In this country, it is called the Chanterelle or occasionally the Golden Chanterelle. Fairly common and easy to spot, the Chanterelle grows in great profusion some years. It is one of just a few mushrooms that are the same color over the entire fruit body. Very beautiful, the Chanterelle has great taste and aroma and is visually appealing when served.

Cap (pileus): The cap measures from three-fourths of an inch to five inches wide and is convex at first with an inrolled margin (cap edge), often becoming funnel-shaped with a wavy margin. It can be quite irregularly shaped. The color ranges from egg-yolk yellow to yellow-orange and rarely has pink tones. The Pink/Peach Chanterelle is called *Cantharellus persicinus* by some mycologists. Older specimens are more likely to be more orange especially after being rained on a few times. Specimens that receive a lot of sun can bleach out toward a whitish color and have a slightly leathery appearance. Because the Chanterelle can persist for two or three weeks, algae may grow on top giving it some greenish tones, which is somewhat common in wet, mossy areas with shade.

29

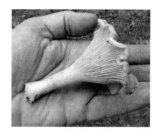
29

Ridges: What look to be gills are actually ridges, which are more like folds or wrinkles that are forked and usually with blunt edges that are the same color as the rest of the mushroom. Often quite wavy and always running down the stem (decurrent), these ridges can be a little sharper-edged and deeper than the description in some field guides might suggest.

Stem (stipe): The length of the stem is usually similar to the width of the cap and about the same color as the rest of the mushroom. Sometimes the stem is a bit whiter.

Flesh: The flesh is yellowish white to white.

Spores: The spore print is whitish to slightly yellow.

When and where to find them (ecology): Chanterelles are mycorrhizal, meaning they form associations with trees and possibly some other bushes or plants. I believe they sometimes associate with mosses, as well; but trees will still be around. If there are no trees, the specimen is not a Chanterelle. A lot of moss is a good indicator some Chanterelles may be around although they may not grow in the moss, but nearby. In the early part of the season starting at the end of June, specimens will be mostly around eastern white pine but other trees may also support them. As the season progresses, Chanterelles can be found under a wide variety of trees, such as oak, hemlock, and balsam fir, birch, beech, and spruce. I have found only one Chanterelle under red maple, numerous specimens in poison ivy, and a few in low-bush blueberries that were fairly near trees. Because Chanterelles can grow for two to three weeks expanding in size greatly, it may be best to leave the smaller specimens for later picking.

Chanterelles can grow in both uplands and lowlands and

can often be found in washes or along trail edges and country dirt roads with mixed woods and a lot of shade. I have always found edges to be interesting. I often come to the edge of a dirt road or trail edge and find groupings or lines of Chanterelles. Although it is easy to imagine that the woods interior will hold many more, often that is not the case. I think the compacted earth of the trail or road may cause the mycelium to react by fruiting.

Fairly bug resistant, a Chanterelle may have a maggot or two once in a while one; but in general, bugs are not present. Slugs may eat Chanterelles. During dry years when there are not as many mushrooms growing, Chanterelles may exhibit more infestation than normal. The fungus gnats probably lay eggs there because they have fewer choices.

July through September are likely to be the biggest months for finding Chanterelles but a few may come up as late as November. Consistent summer rains tend to produce bountiful growth.

Preparation: The Chanterelle is truly delicious when sautéed but is not that tasty as tempura. As a dried product, the Chanterelle does not reconstitute well for cooking but makes a great powder for seasoning when used in small quantity or for flavoring when used in larger quantity. Chanterelle powder added to alfredo or a béchamel-based (white) sauce is truly outstanding. Best used with foods that are associated with white wine, the powder's flavor subtleties make it suited for plain preparation or served with chicken, veal, pork, fish, milder-flavored vegetables, rice, pasta, potatoes, nuts, or fruits. Sautéed Chanterelles may be finished with cream for an easy but elegant sauce. Mixing with strong-flavored foods is not recommended. It is not the right mushroom for steak. Chanterelles are best not mixed with the overpowering flavor of the White Button Mushroom.

If you have the luxury of having enough Chanterelles to make powder, you can make Chanterelle-flavored vinegar, oil, or liquor. Mushroom powder is strong stuff. It is likely to impart two or three times more flavor than reconstituted dried whole mushrooms.

Comments: Some say that Chanterelles smell like apricots. I consider this opinion a stretch, but they do have a fruity, perfume-like aroma that becomes very noticeable if they are in a bag or closed container for a few minutes. To me, it is Chanterelle aroma. Chanterelles can have a mildly peppery taste. I noticed the peppery character when I made some Chanterelle liquor.

In the west the prevailing species is *Cantharellus formosus.* It was previously lumped in with our eastern Chanterelle as *Cantharellus cibarius* but now the western species has its own epithet. It does have a slightly different look in that it is larger, chunkier, and often has some pinkish tones especially on the ridges.

Chanterelles can look somewhat like the poisonous Jack O'Lantern. The Jack O'Lantern has sharp-edged gills and pumpkin orange color growing in dense bunches with many stems joined at the base (cespitose). Chanterelles also look somewhat like the so-called False Chanterelle *(Hygrophoropsis aurantica).* False Chanterelles have a feltlike (finely tomentose) cap, close sharp-edged gills, thinner stems, orange-brown tones, and may not be the same color all over the fruit body the way Chanterelles are. False Chanterelles are not fragrant. Some say they

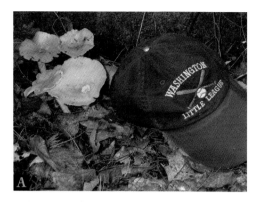

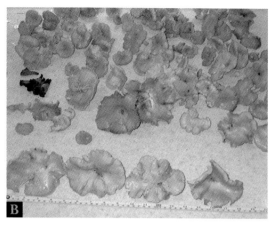

Figure A: Extra large mature Chanterelles. **Figure B:** Four extra large Chanterelles measuring nineteen inches. **Figure C:** Occasionally Chanterelles can have a pink tint. The Pink/Peach Chanterelle is called *Cantharellus persicinus* by some mycologists. **Figure D:** Chanterelles may be joined like this.

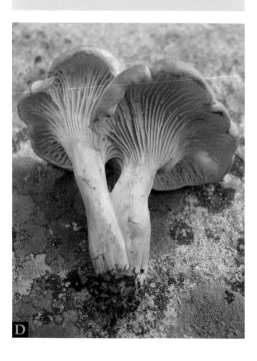

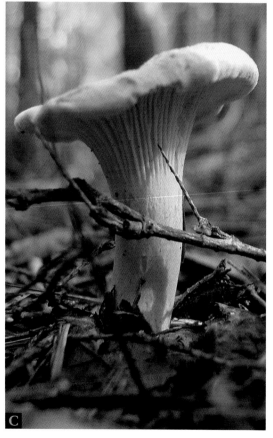

are mildly poisonous while others regard them as merely a culinary disappointment. Do *not* eat False Chanterelles.

Chanterelles can be used for dyeing wool, some fabrics, and paper. When ammonia is used as a mordant, *Cantharellus cibarius* will yield a muted yellow color with wool.

Jack O'Lantern
(Omphalotus illudens)

Known as the Chanterelle look-alike, the Jack O'Lantern is poisonous. Once you have positively identified Chanterelles, you should never make a mistake with these two species. Side by side, they do not look that much alike. Chanterelles *never* grow in the ways pictured below.

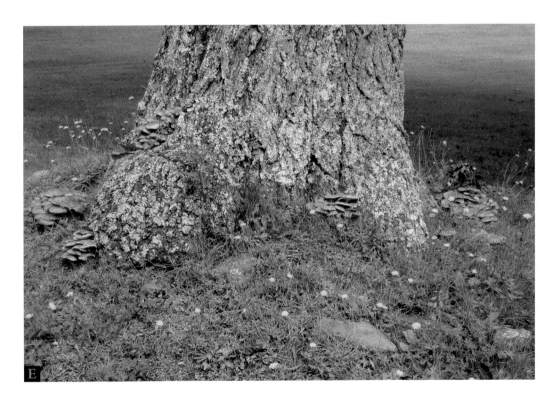

Figure E: Jack O'Lantern grows in large bunches with stems attached together at the base (cespitose). The bunches are often large and found below oak and other hardwood trees. Sometimes they are found in a lawn where there is buried wood or roots. Chanterelles do not grow this way—ever. Figure F: The Jack O'Lantern is quite poisonous and should not be confused with the Chanterelle. Jack O'Lantern are usually fairly large with a two-and-one-half- to four-inch cap and can be much larger. Most specimens will be of similar size. Chanterelles, however, *never* grow this way. Figure G: The Scaly Vase Chanterelle *(Gomphus floccosus)* is not a true Chanterelle. It is very dense with a scaly orange cap. Although some eat this species, the Scaly Vase Chanterelle is quite indigestible, mildly toxic to many people, and should be avoided. Figure H: The Jack O'Lantern has sharp-edged gills and pumpkin orange color. Whereas, Chanterelles have blunt-edged, forked, and often wavy gills that tend to run down the stem more. Chanterelles are quite variable in size and usually more yellow color. The specimen on the right is a mature Chanterelle.

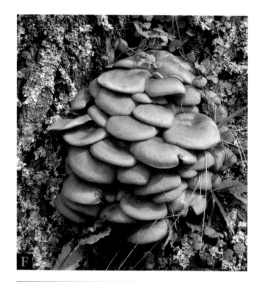

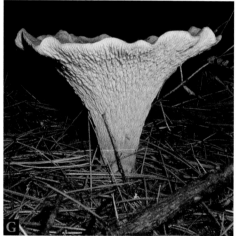

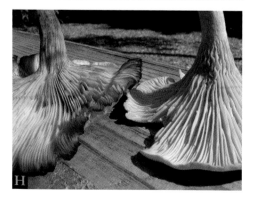

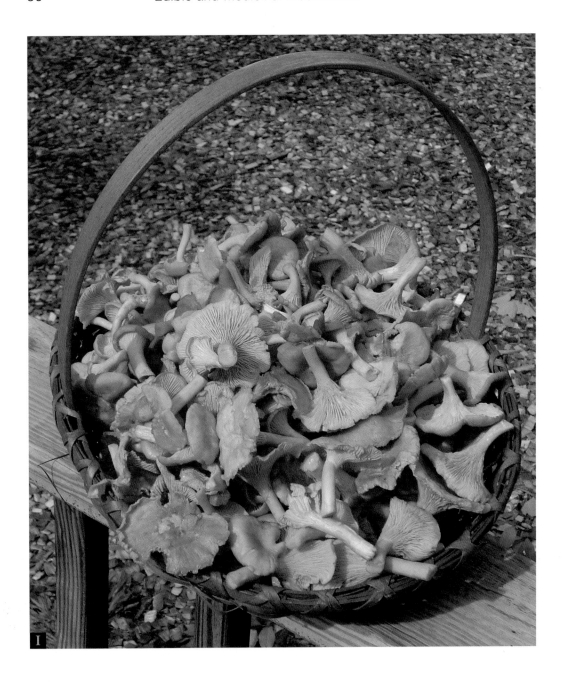

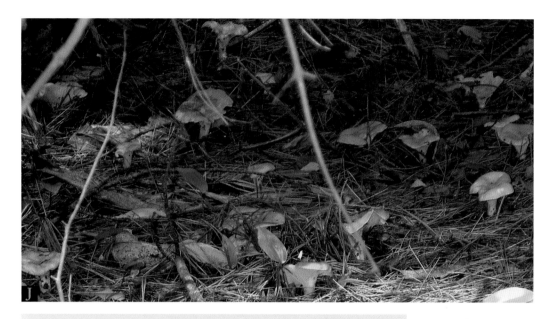

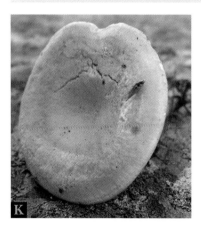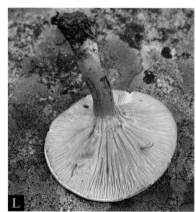

Figure I: The year 2006 was very rainy and the biggest year for Chanterelles I have ever seen. There were exceptionally large stands with large fruit in mixed woods. **Figure J:** Chanterelles when found in large groups are going to be spread about (gregarious) as seen here under a balsam fir. **Figure K:** False Chanterelles (*Hygrophoropsis aurantical*) have close sharp-edged gills, thinner stems, a feltlike (finely tomentose) cap, and often orange-brown tones (above and right). Do *not* eat False Chanterelles. **Figure L:** Note the brownish stem on this False Chanterelle.

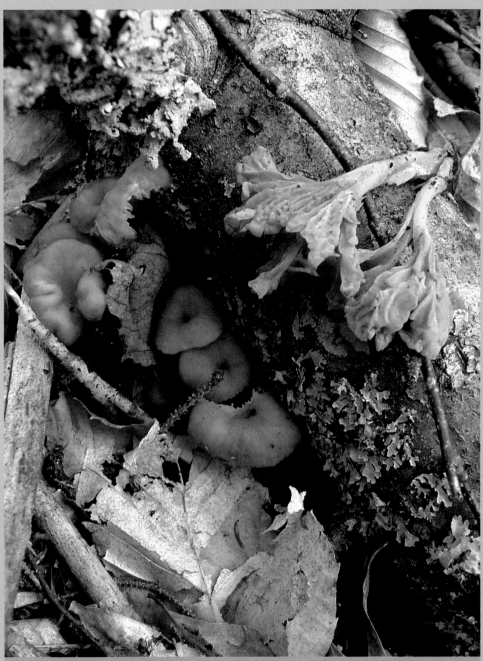

Craterellus ignicolor is known by some as Yellow Foot Chanterelle
and Flame-colored Chanterelle.

Chapter Three

Small Chanterelles

(Craterellus tubaeformis and C. ignicolor)

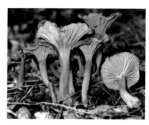

Craterellus tubae-formis is also called the Winter Chanterelle.

There are smaller, more delicate "chanterelles" that grow throughout the summer and into the fall. They have a similar look to Chanterelles with their shape and the blunt-edged, gill-like ridges that run partway down the stem. The semi-hollow and funnel-like shape suggests the two species are halfway between a Chanterelle and a Black Trumpet. Unlike Chanterelles, *Craterellus tubaeformis* and *C. ignicolor* tend to grow in clusters. Taxonomy is in transition within the Cantharellus and Craterellus genus. The two species were previously classified in the *Cantharellus* genus, but DNA study has placed them in the closely related *Craterellus* genus or clade. The various small "chanterelles" may be a challenge to figure out for taxonomists, but these closely related species all seem to be edible and good. I suspect that these species are saprobic rather than mycorrhizal as they are often found on or near very dead wood.

Cap (pileus): The cap (pileus) ranges from three-fourths of an inch wide to two and one-half inches wide for both species. Funnel-shaped and considerably more delicate than *Cantharellus cibarius,* the Golden Chanterelle, *Craterellus tubaeformis* has a yellowish brown or brown funnel-shaped cap. *C. ignicolor* looks very similar but is yellow-orange.

Ridges: The blunt, forked, and often wavy gill-like ridges that run partway down the stem are quite shallow and usually look like veins or wrinkles. *Craterellus tubaeformis* has gray or violet-gray blunt ridges descending the stem. *C. ignicolor* has yellow-orange ridges that descend the stem.

Stem (stipe): The stem of both species is yellow-orange developing hollowness with age. *Craterellus tubaeformis* often has slightly brown tones.

Flesh: *Craterellus tubaeformis* flesh is brownish yellow, and *C. ignicolor* is orange-yellow.

Spores: Both species make a whitish spore print.

When and where to find them (ecology): From August to November these can be found around similar locations of hardwoods and mixed woods, especially where dead wood, wood chips, or thick duff is present. *Craterellus tubaeformis* tends to appear a bit later than *C. ignicolor.* Sphagnum-type mosses are often present. More likely to be in clusters than *Cantharellus cibarius,* both *Craterellus tubaeformis* and *C. ignicolor* are quite common and can be an indicator that Black Trumpets are nearby. The aroma signature of *Craterellus tubaeformis* and *C. ignicolor* is quite similar to the Chanterelle. If you place *Craterellus tubaeformis* and *C. ignicolor* in a closed bag for a few minutes and then open it, you will smell a beautiful perfume-like, fruity aroma that some say is similar to apricots. Smelling only remotely like apricots to me, their aroma is indeed distinctive and quite pleasant.

Preparation: Try only a little the first time. The aroma when drying *Craterellus tubaeformis* and *C. ignicolor* is outstanding.

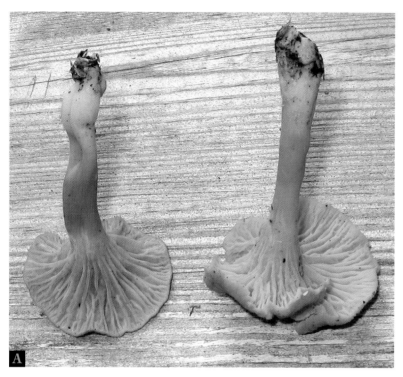

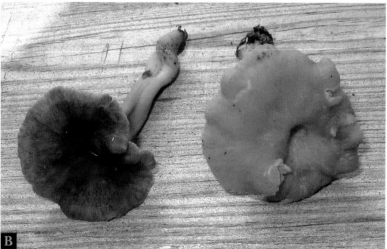

❧ **Figure A:** *Craterellus tubaeformis* is shown on the left and *C. igni-color* is on the right. ❧ **Figure B:** These images compare *Craterellus tubaeformis* and *Craterellus ignicolor.*

They can be sautéed for truly great flavor but are far less interesting when deep-fried. Simple preparation is often the best way to showcase their subtle flavor. They reconstitute well and make a nice mushroom powder that is outstanding for flavoring alfredo and béchamel-based sauces. Because the flavor is subtle, it should only be mixed in certain ways. A *Cantharellus-Craterellus* mix is nice. I consider these "white wine" mushrooms. Chicken, pork, fish, rice, pasta, as well as vegetables and soups are good choices for recipes using these.

Comments: There is a lot of confusion around *Craterellus tubaeformis* and *Craterellus ignicolor.* They are often seen listed as *Cantharellus tubaeformis* or *Cantharellus ignicolor.* DNA studies have determined that both species are actually part of the *Craterellus* genus. *Craterellus tubaeformis* and *C. infundibuliformis* have been determined to be the same species although many field guides list them as separate species. Sometimes you will find listings for *Cantharellus xanthopus* that is extremely similar to *Craterellus ignicolor.* Hopefully, the DNA of these closely related species will be sorted out soon. As with all edible mushrooms tried for the first time, just try a little at first. All the small, confusing "Chanterelles" seem to be edible.

Craterellus tubaeformis and *C. ignicolor* can be used for dyeing textiles and paper. When ammonia is used as a mordant, both species will yield a muted yellow color with wool.

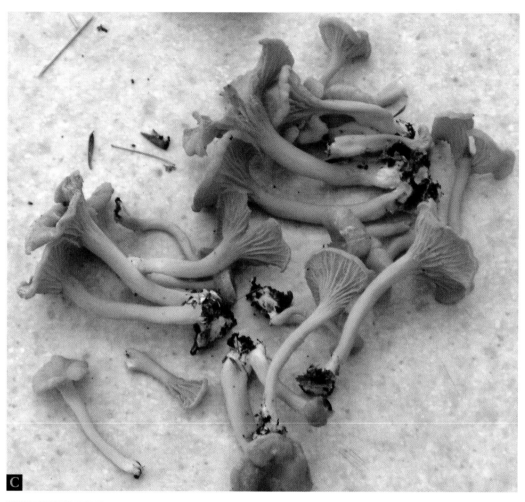

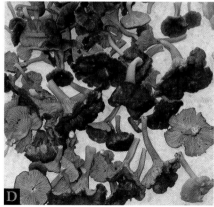

🌱 **Figure C:** *Craterellus ignicolor.* 🌱 **Figure D:** *Craterellus tubaeformis.*

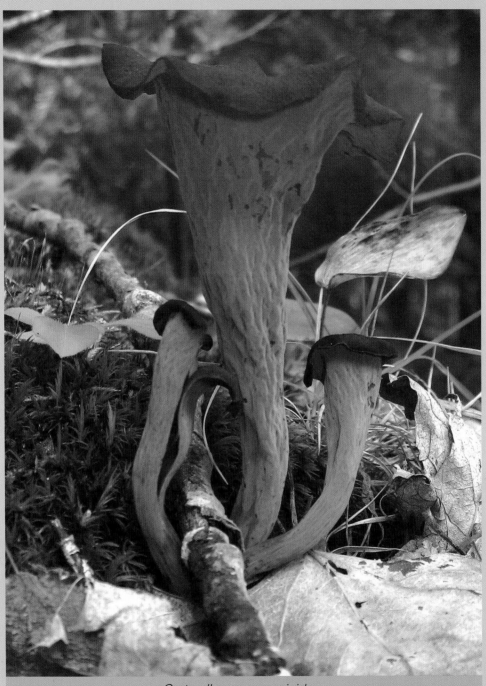
Craterellus cornucopioides.

Chapter Four

Black Trumpets

(Craterellus cornucopioides, C. cinereus, and *C. foetidus)*

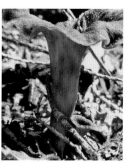

Appearance and color can vary quite a bit between Black Trumpets, but their taste is always the absolute best.

D uring the years that I have collected mushrooms, I mostly made my own way, not joining clubs or forays. I barely knew they existed. In the 1970s and '80s, I stayed relatively conservative in my approach to collecting—only adding a species to my edible list once or twice a year. Occasionally I saw a few Black Trumpets but did not pick or eat them. Then after I first tried them a few years ago, I realized I had been missing possibly the best-tasting mushroom of all. When I first started looking for Black Trumpets, I found nothing. It was not until this past year when I learned how to find a lot. I also learned that there are at least four distinct types of "trumpets" in this area.

It is all about how one directs his or her attention. My collecting style worked fine for Chanterelles and other more obvious mushrooms, because I was always trying to see from a distance rather than looking straight down. I was always spotting trees from a distance. This strategy will not work for finding Black Trumpets because they cannot be spotted from a distance.

The various Black Trumpets are all funnel-shaped and gray, brown, or black; they often grow in small bunches and occasionally singly; and they range in height from one to six inches.

Cap (pileus): The cap measures from three-fourths of an inch to three inches across with very thin flesh. It is gray, brown, or black with a flowerlike appearance except for *Craterellus foetidus,* which has a flatter, thicker, grayer, and more Chanterelle-like cap. All have a very strong perfume-like aroma. Very fragrant, Black Trumpets smell stronger than any other type of mushroom I have found.

Gills: Gills are not present in *Craterellus cornucopioides;* instead, the surface will be smooth or have just the slightest hint of ridges and be black, brown, or rust color. *C. foetidus* and *C. cinereus* have shallow, gray gill ridges.

Stem (stipe): The stem is hollow in all types and very thin except for *Craterellus foetidus,* which has a thicker, somewhat meaty stem.

Flesh: The flesh is gray, brown, or black and very thin. *Craterellus foetidus* has slightly thicker gray flesh.

Spores: The spore print is white to pinkish.

When and where to find them (ecology): Jerry Goguen from Massachusetts came to Maine in 2006 and we went on a mushroom walk in a wildlife management area in Hallowell. He gave me Black Trumpet lessons. He explained to me about washes—which are intermittent streams on hills, on small mountains, and in valleys where water rushes through during spring runoff and heavy rainstorms. Sometimes the water creates natural "dams" of dead trees or branches that fall and are washed down the hill and lodge sideways behind living trees. A stone wall can also be a "dam." Black Trumpets and Chanterelles tend to proliferate in washes below these dams especially in the presence of moss, beeches, and mixed woods. Washes can often be followed long distances with phenomenal results.

In order to spot these species, you have to look directly down. In this area of Maine, Black Trumpets like the beech and oak trees and growing on hummocks underneath the trees or nearby. Trumpets look similar to brown, black, or gray pansies growing among leaves and other natural camouflage so it is important to pay attention to your surroundings. These species tend to grow in the same places year after year.

Trumpets come in late June and continue through the summer. Beeches, mixed woods, as well as low, shady, and damp locations—such as ponds and swamps—are good places to look. I found a very small variety under hemlock. They seemed to have slightly less flavor than the others but were still very good. The four *Craterellus* species I have found were delicious.

Preparation: As always, just taste a few if it is your first time. Black Trumpets are highly aromatic and flavorful. They are delicious when sautéed, tempura-fried, or dried. I think they are best plainly prepared or in a recipe that showcases their flavor. Trumpets need to be very carefully cleaned. Their trumpet shape may capture quite a bit of sand, dirt, or other vegetable matter. Sometimes splitting them in half is best. You can easily do this by gently pulling at opposite sides of the cap.

Trumpets are best mixed with species that have similar flavor characteristics, like various species of *Craterellus* and *Cantharellus*. Milder-flavored wild species, like Shaggy Mane, Chicken of the Woods, or the similar-flavored Hedgehogs will also mix with Black Trumpets. Foods associated with white wine, such as seafood, chicken, veal, pork, rice, pasta, cheese and certain sauces, blend well with Black Trumpets. They have a stronger flavor signature that lends itself to more culinary experimentation. For example, at the 2006 Maine Mycological Association annual meeting, mycologist Greg Marley presented a Black Trumpet white pizza that was scrumptious.

Author and mushroom expert David Fischer of American-Mushrooms.com suggests using Black Trumpets to flavor white wine. I tried it and found it to be very pleasant

Comments: Recent DNA studies suggest that *Craterellus cornucopioides* and *C. fallax* are the same mushroom even though they have slightly different looks and spore print colors. Eventu-

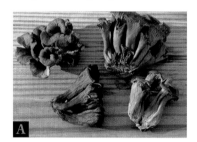

ally, DNA analysis may sort out the taxonomic confusion. Every type of *Craterellus* I have tried has been absolutely delicious.

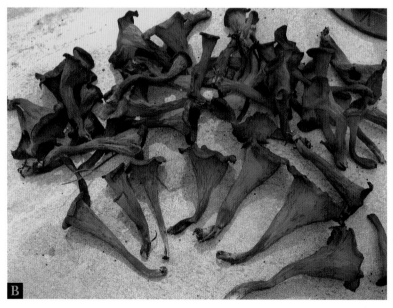

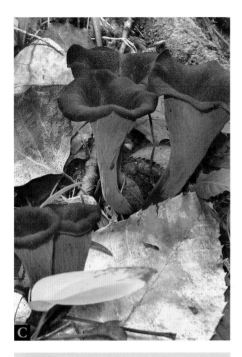

C

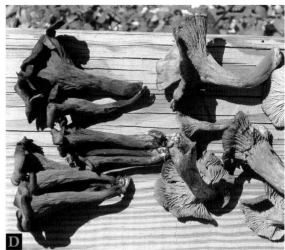

D

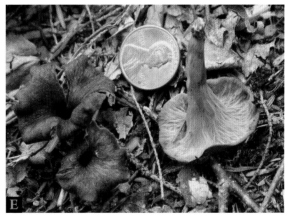

E

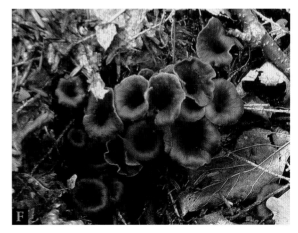

F

⚕ **Figure A:** Shown on the right are a form of Trumpets that I believe are *Craterellus cinereus,* on the left are *Craterellus cornucopioides.* ⚕ **Figure B:** An example of a productive afternoon of collecting. ⚕ **Figure C:** *Craterellus cornucopioides.* ⚕ **Figure D:** On the right are a gray form of Trumpets with discernable ridges that I believe are *Craterellus foetidus;* on the left are *Craterellus cornucopioides.* ⚕ **Figure E:** Fortunately, there were more than enough of these little *Craterellus calyculus* for a substantial meal. ⚕ **Figure F:** *Craterellus calyculus.*

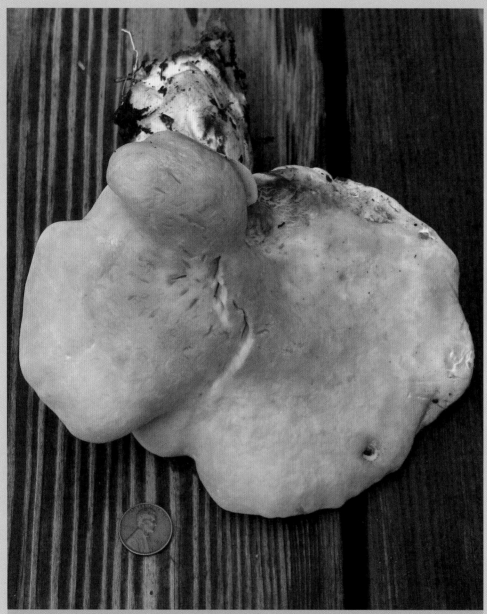

Top view of *Hydnum repandum*.

Chapter Five

Hedgehog Mushrooms

(Hydnum repandum and *H. umbilicatum)*

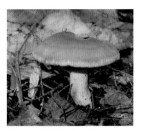

Hydnum
umbilicatum.

There are two closely related species of Hedgehog Mushrooms, which are also known as Sweet Tooth Mushrooms: *Hydnum repandum* and *H. umbilicatum.* Both have teeth rather than gills or pores making them quite easy mushrooms to identify. They are close relatives of the Chanterelle and the aroma of *Hydnum repandum* and *H. umbilicatum* is strikingly similar. Both species can often be found in profusion beginning in midsummer and continuing into late fall. Fortunately, insects and slugs tend to leave these species alone, which can be refreshing during the summer because so many good-looking mushrooms can be infested during the warmer months.

Cap (pileus): The cap of *Hydnum repandum* ranges from two to eight inches wide, thick, and usually convex but often irregularly shaped with lobes. Occasionally the cap of *H. repandum* will become flat or upturned and usually have a wavy margin. Color varies from cream to orangey brown. H. repandum may develop an orangey color when bruised. The cap of *Hydnum umbilicatum* is usually orangey brown with a sunken depression on top above where the stem joins the cap. In addition, the cap of *H. umbilicatum* is considerably smaller and has a more centered stem than *H. repandum.*

Teeth: Rather than gills or pores, both species have whitish to light brown toothlike structures between one-eighth and one-fourth inches long that break off very easily. *Hydnum umbilicatum* teeth are usually a somewhat darker color than *H. repandum*.

Stem (stipe): The stem of *Hydnum repandum* is short and thick and is usually off center and often irregularly shaped. *H. umbilicatum* has a thinner, longer, and more-centered stem.

Flesh: The flesh of *Hydnum repandum* is thick, whitish, and stains slightly orange when cut or bruised. Whereas, *H. umbilicatum* has thin, whitish flesh that does not stain.

Spores: Both species make a white spore print.

When and where to find them (ecology): *Hydnum repandum* is usually found around hardwoods, such as birch and beech. A very mature yellow birch very near my home produces a substantial harvest most years. Usually *H. repandum* starts showing in August and can continue into early November in mixed woods. *H. umbilicatum* is usually found under conifers and in wetter areas during the same time span but mostly in September and October. If you discover one specimen, you will often find dozens. Last fall while looking for Matsutake, I stopped next to a stand of hemlocks near a lake that looked promising to me. There I found a piece of black thread tied to a bush near the side of the road that led into the woods to a hemlock grove in the interior. I could see that this thread led to someone's secret Matsutake stand. Unfortunately, I was too late and could see the holes around the hemlocks where they had been picked. With a little looking around, though, I found more than a hundred *H. umbilicatum* that the Matsutake hunter had overlooked.

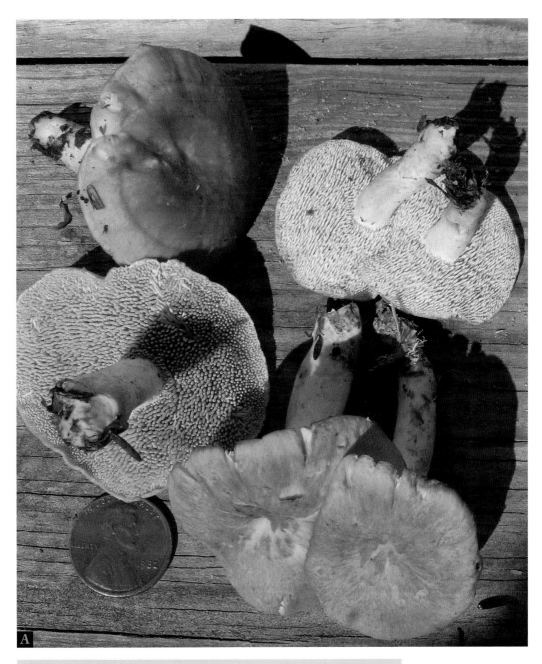

🦔 **Figure A:** *Hydnum umbilicatum.*

Preparation: Both of these species can be prepared in similar fashion. They are white wine mushrooms that are nice sautéed, fried, and dried. Both have a crunchy but not chewy texture. The flavor and smell is somewhat similar to Chanterelles. Being much larger and thicker, *Hydnum repandum* can be used in more ways than Chanterelles including microwave. The bigger, chunkier *H. repandum* also fries quite successfully. When drying Hedgehogs, the aroma is wonderful; in fact, I do not think any mushroom makes my house smell better. Neither species reconstitutes very well so making a mushroom powder from either may be the best use.

Comments: Both species are delicious and not that hard to find during the warmer summer months, when many other species are bug infested. The teeth make Hedgehogs easy to identify.

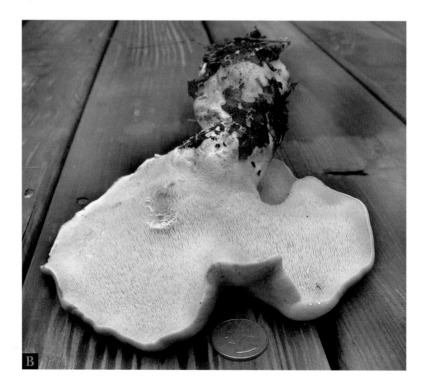

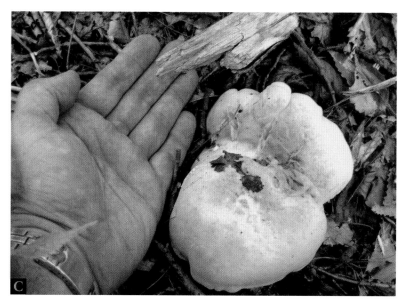

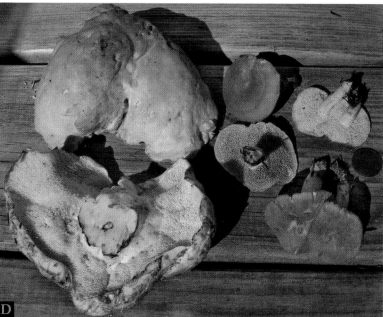

❧ **Figure B:** Bottom view of *Hydnum repandum*. ❧ **Figure C:** *Hydnum repandum*. ❧ **Figure D:** *Hydnum repandum* is on the left and *H. umbilicatum* is on the right.

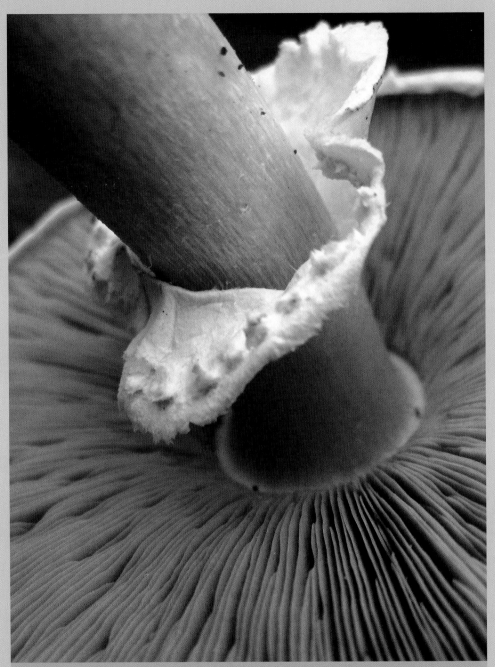

Close view of *Agaricus arvensis* stem with the pebbly, hanging veil and the grayish pink free gills, which will later change to dark brown with age.

Chapter Six

Horse Mushroom and Meadow Mushroom

(Agaricus arvensis and *A. campestris)*

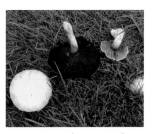

These Meadow Mushrooms were in front of a bank in weedless grass, suggesting herbicide usage thus rendering them unsuitable for consumption.

Summer is the beginning of the season for two species of *Agaricus,* the Horse Mushroom *(Agaricus arvensis)* and the Meadow Mushroom *(A. campestris).* These species are closely related to the White Button/Cremini/Portobello Mushrooms you find in the supermarket. The Meadow Mushroom usually appears in lawns, pastures, and open areas. It is similar in size to the White Button Mushroom but not as thick and dense. The Horse Mushroom is usually quite large—often larger than the biggest Portobello caps you may purchase. The *A. arvensis* is a species with big flavor. In Maine, they seem to grow especially well in coastal locations.

Fruit body: Horse Mushrooms range in color from white to slightly tannish or yellowish and often have long stems with a hanging textured veil. The caps have fairly obvious scales and are very regular in shape. The edge of the cap (margin) often has veil remnants making it slightly ragged. By comparison, Meadow Mushrooms have whiter smooth caps of a less regular shape, usually smaller scales, and a shorter stem that often tapers at the base. Veil remnants are seen on the stem of the Meadow Mushroom but only occasionally on the cap margin.

Cap (pileus): The cap of the Horse Mushroom (*Agaricus arvensis*) measures from four to twelve inches wide. The cap is white at first but turns slightly yellowish tan as it matures with a slightly brownish patch at top center and some slight scaliness. As the cap is about to open, it can be round and as big as a softball mimicking a Puffball. As the cap starts to open, the veil spreads fairly wide and have a circle of pebbly warts finally breaking away, leaving a large hanging veil on the stem and a ragged edge at the edge of the cap (margin). Horse Mushrooms have an anise / almond aroma that is quite strong and exceptionally pleasant. The flesh of the cap or stem of *A. arvensis* may bruise very slightly yellow. The cap of the Meadow Mushroom *(A. campestris)* is one to five inches wide, whitish, and smooth. The shape can be somewhat wavy and irregular. It may stain slightly pink when handled or waterlogged.

Gills (lamellae): Both species have sharp-edged, close, free gills (not attached to the stem). In immature unopened specimens of *Agaricus arvensis,* the gills are grayish cream. Shortly after the veil breaks, the gills are pinkish, then they change to brown and almost black by the time they mature. If a specimen has white gills, throw it out immediately!

Stem (stipe): The stem of *Agaricus arvensis* is between three and ten inches tall, one-half to one inch thick, mostly smooth above the veil, somewhat scaly below the veil, and thicker at the base. There is no cup at the base as with the poisonous *Amanita.* The stem of a Horse Mushroom will usually have a long hanging veil with pebbly warts at the edge that eventually may come off leaving a ring. Dryness will cause the veil to wrinkle and recede or even to fall off. The flesh may stain very slightly yellow. The base of the stem is not yellow.

The stem of the Meadow Mushroom *(Agaricus campestris)* is from one to four inches tall, whitish to light brown, often tapers to be thinner at the base, usually has just a ring or slight veil remnants, and is somewhat scaly above the veil. The stem and flesh may stain slightly pink. There is no cup at the base of the stem.

Flesh: The flesh of both species is whitish, fairly thick, and similar in density to the White Button Mushroom from the store. Both have an almond/anise scent. Horse Mushrooms usually have a stronger aroma and do not absorb water easily, whereas Meadow Mushrooms can absorb quite a bit of water making them a bit softer and turning the flesh pinkish to brownish.

Spores: The spore prints of both species are dark brown.

When and where to find them: Horse Mushrooms appear usually in September and sometimes continue well into November. I hunt coastal areas but often find them other places as well. Lawns, fields, and pastures are the best places to look. Occasionally specimens can be found around spruce or other conifers, especially if there is grass nearby. Horse Mushrooms tend to like rich soil often with a manure component. Places in lawns where the grass is quite a bit greener and longer are places specimens may soon appear in rings or long lines. Because of their size and abundance, I have picked two bushels in less than five minutes in some places.

Meadow Mushrooms may appear as early as July and may continue into November in lawns, pastures, and open areas. *Agaricus campestris* can be in fairy rings on lawns where the grass is greener and longer. Inside a fairy ring is the mycelium

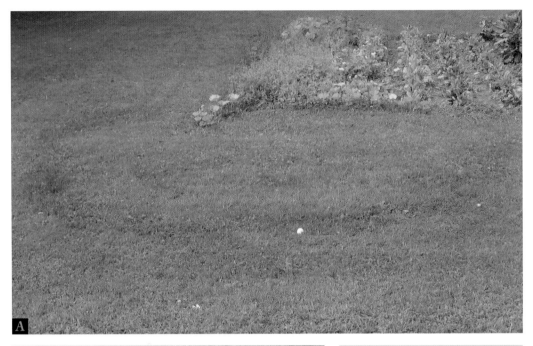

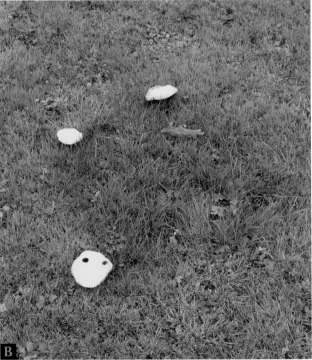

Figure A: This shows a ring of greener, taller grass where a fairy ring of *Agaricus campestris* is growing just to the outside of the dark ring. The substrate inside the ring is likely used up so the underground mycelium moves outward forming a ring. There were two rings in this yard. **Figure B:** This patch of *Agaricus campestris* may form a larger ring next year.

that is consuming organic matter in the soil and pushing outward. Nitrogen is created at the outer part of the ring, causing
the grass to become greener and the mycelium to fruit at the
edge. The ring becomes a few inches larger each year.

Both Horse and Meadow Mushrooms tend to grow in the
same places year after year. They are occasionally found in
very close proximity to each other. Because we have had
weather fluctuating between wet and dry with long periods
of dryness in Maine for three years, I have not found as many
specimens.

Preparation: These species are an excellent complement with
many foods and wines. Having a strong flavor, Horse and Meadow Mushrooms lend themselves to most cooking processes.
It best to cook them soon after you pick them to capture their
strong anise/almond aroma that can dissipate somewhat after
short storage. Tempura is a great technique for retaining this
anise/almond character. The more mature the two species
become, the stronger their flavor. They are excellent sautéed,
as tempura, microwaved, dried, in soup, grilled, stuffed, and
so forth. Both are great with steak and other strong-flavored
red meat. Because of their versatility, use them in many
recipes. They are also far superior in flavor to the *Agaricus bisporus* available at the supermarket. The flavor of Horse and
Meadow Mushrooms will never be lost in a mix but certainly
may overpower.

Specimens that fill the entire frying pan are easily possible.
I once found a fourteen-inch Horse Mushroom cap! I often
cook the big caps whole and freeze them with layers of plastic wrap between them so you can take out one at a time during the winter. They do freeze well after cooking, and this is

often necessary because you frequently find much more than you can consume right away. A large Horse Mushroom cap can be used as "dough" for pizza, placing pizza sauce or salsa on the cap and then adding other meat, vegetables, cheese, and other toppings. One thing to note with mature caps is that a lot of spores will come out and you will have a dark brown juice in your pan, which can seriously darken or discolor foods you add it to. This can be a good thing for gravy; but the juice will turn light sauces—such as béchamel, alfredo, or Mornay—brown, and they will look far less appealing.

Smaller than Horse Mushrooms, Meadow Mushrooms are somewhat less versatile because their size, thickness, and water absorbency. They soak up liquid readily. Horse Mushrooms do not absorb water into the flesh easily. I often make slurries by placing the caps of both species in water to soak out the spores for distribution outdoors. Meadow Mushrooms readily sponge water up and will eventually sink. Whereas, the gills of Horse Mushrooms will take on water but still float like a cork even after a couple of days of soaking.

Comments: Both species are strong tasting and usable in most recipes in which you would use White Button Mushrooms from the supermarket. The flavor is superior to the supermarket offerings. Try only a small bit the first time. Mature specimens of *Agaricus arvensis* and *A. campestris* make a heavy brown spore print within minutes. They *never* have white gills when open or a white or green spore print! *Agaricus silvicola* looks practically identical to *A. arvensis* but *A. silvicola* is usually found in conifer woods. It is usually more slender. It is a choice edible. The poisonous *Agaricus xanthodermis* is a similar species with a phenolic odor (like creosote) and yellowish base, which stains or bruises bright yellow. Any bad smelling or strongly yellow staining *Agaricus* should be avoided. A Horse Mushroom may occasionally stain very slightly yellow but *not* a strong chrome yellow.

Horse and Meadow Mushrooms can be used for dyeing wool, some fabrics, and paper. Wool will become a yellow-tan color when salt water is used as a mordant or a gray-green color when cooked in an iron pot.

It may be possible to get Horse and Meadow Mushrooms to grow in your lawn by making a slurry from your rejected specimens to extract spores or by putting the caps in a place you think would be suitable. I have tried it with both species.

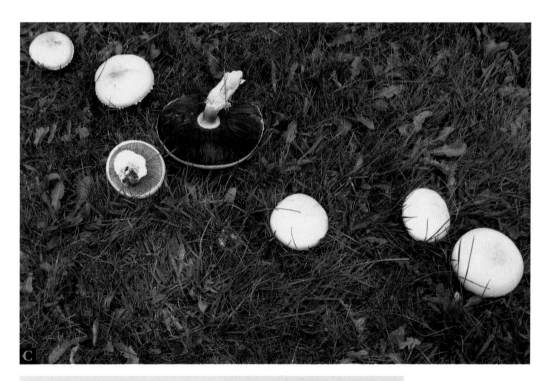

Figure C: Weeds in the grass suggests that herbicides were not used here and these Horse Mushrooms would be a safe, choice edible.

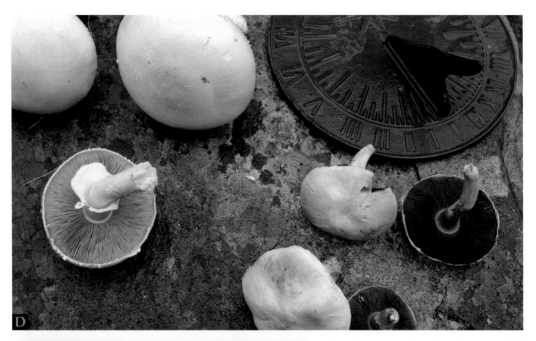

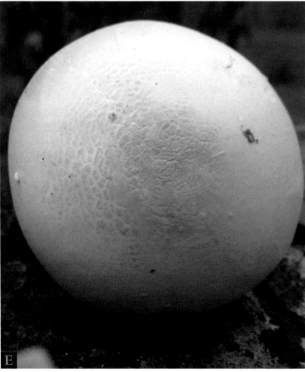

Figure D: Here is a comparison of Horse Mushroom (*Agaricus arvensis*) on the left and Meadow Mushroom (*A. campestris*) on the right. The *A. arvensis* are somewhat younger with pinker gills than the *A. campestris,* which is commonly known as Pink Bottoms. These specimens were collected on the same day less than two hundred feet apart after heavy rain. The Meadow Mushrooms absorbed water and were heavy. The Horse Mushrooms were lighter and dry. **Figure E:** This is a close-up of the *Agaricus arvensis* with its regular shape, tannish center, and slightly scaly cap.

❧ **Figure F:** *Agaricus arvensis* is on the left and *A. campestris* on the right. Note the slightly ragged veil remnants at the edge (margin) of the cap of *A. arvensis*. *A. campestris* stem is shorter and often tapers to be thinner at the base. *A. arvensis* stem tends to be bulbous at the base and longer. There is no cup at the base. ❧ **Figure G:** *Agaricus arvensis* is on the left and *A. campestris* on the right. *A. campestris* is whiter, smoother, and less regular in shape. *A. campestris* shows slight pink bruising on the cap, probably from rainwater and handling. ❧ **Figure H:** Note the less regular shape of the cap on these *Agaricus campestris* and some pinkish tones from rainwater and handling. These specimens are somewhat waterlogged. ❧ **Figure I:** *Agaricus campestris* with veil remnants, tapering stem, and pinkish brown free gills, which will change to dark brown later.

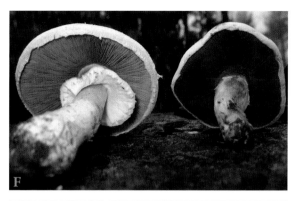

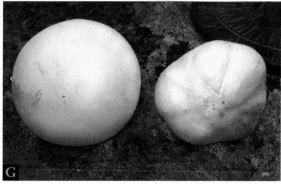

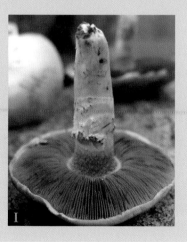

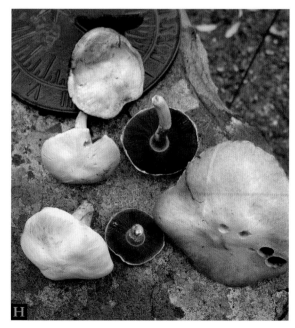

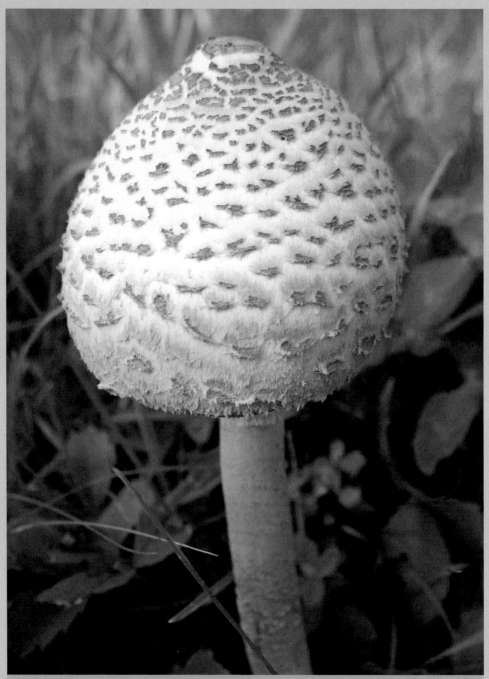

Parasol Mushroom *(Macrolepiota procera)*.

Chapter Seven

Parasol Mushroom
(Macrolepiota procera)

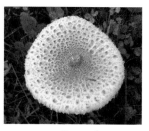

Parasol Mushroom *(Macrolepiota procera).*

The Parasol Mushroom *(Macrolepiota procera)*, formerly known as *Lepiota procera,* has exceptionally fine flavor. This species should not be collected until you are extremely confident of your identification skills. The Parasol is not that hard to identify, but you *must* be exceptionally observant of all characteristics because there are some *Lepiota* relatives that are very poisonous or even deadly. You also cannot make the mistake of collecting *Amanitas,* which can also be poisonous or deadly. Be sure to consult your field guides and if possible check with a local expert. Always make a spore print, and *never* eat small *Lepiotas* or any with green aspects to the gills or a green spore print.

Fruit body: The Parasol has a broad, scaly, brownish cap with a bulbous-based, tall, scaly, brownish stem. The veil becomes a movable ring that slides up and down the stem.

Cap (pileus): The cap of the *Macrolepiota procera* is egg-shaped and becomes bell-shaped then nearly flat. The cap ranges from three to ten inches wide with attached scales in a regular pattern and a central knob that is brown at first but cracks with age, revealing the white flesh. A mature cap may smell of maple syrup.

Gills (lamellae): The gills of the Parasol Mushroom are broad, rough-edged, white, close, and free.

Stem (stipe): The stem ranges from three to twelve or more inches tall and three-eighths to five eighths of an inch thick. Enlarged to bulbous at the base with brown scales that have a pattern somewhat resemble herringbone. The partial veil becomes a ring that slides up and down the stem.

Flesh: The Parasol has white, moderately thick, and nonbruising flesh.

Spores: The spore print is white.

When and where to find them (ecology): The Parasol Mushroom may be found on lawns, along edges of trails or woods edges, and in the woods. The *Macrolepiota procera* may or may not be near trees although it can have a preference for certain trees. Oak, white pine, or other conifers are often productive places to look, but this species can be in any mixed woods, as well. Large specimens are often found on lawns sometimes in large quantities and may be up to one foot tall.

Preparation: This is a truly delicious tasting mushroom! The mature caps can have the odor and taste of maple syrup. The maple character seems to become more pronounced if it dries just slightly. The Parasol is wonderful sautéed and tempura-fried. This species is best served alone or in a way that showcases its outstanding flavor, such as in a soup or mild sauce. The stems are often discarded because they are tough and fibrous. I suspect they might be used as a duxelles if very finely chopped. I have yet to harvest enough specimens to experiment as much as I would like.

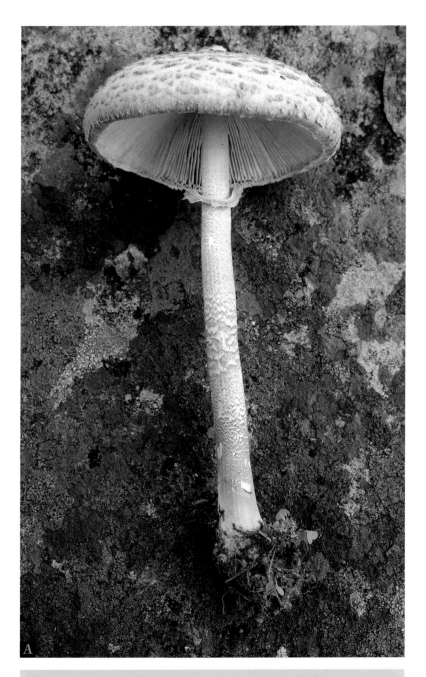

🪶 Figure A: Note the enlarged base of this *Macrolepiota procera* that does not grow from a cup or sac.

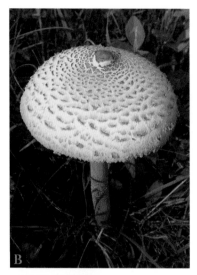

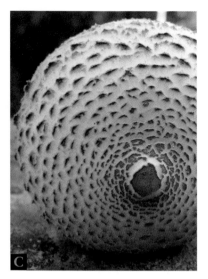

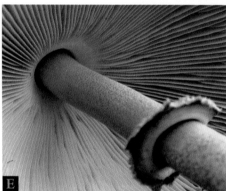

Figure B: Note the protrusion at the center of the cap. **Figure C:** The cap of this *Macrolepiota procera* has attached scales in a regular pattern and a central knob that is brown at first but cracks with age revealing the white flesh. **Figure D:** The gills and margin of a Parasol Mushroom. **Figure E:** The partial veil of this Parasol Mushroom becomes a ring that slides up and down the stem.

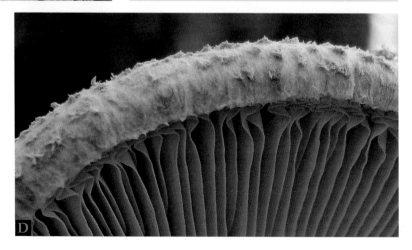

Comments: Be sure to eat just a bit at first to make sure you have no reaction. *Never* consume very small *Lepiotas* or any with any hint of green gills or a green spore print, like *Chlorophyllum molybdites,* which can grow in similar locations and bear a passing resemblance. *C. molybdites* only show greenish gills with age, otherwise they are white. You cannot take chances with this one so you must be absolutely sure or consult a mycologist or experienced mushroomer.

You may have luck making a slurry for propagating the Parasol in your lawn: Place your older or wormy caps in water for a day or so to capture the spores in solution. Then pour the water on your lawn. Of course, if you do this, *never* use weed killer on your lawn.

Other edible larger-sized relatives of the *Macrolepiota procera* are the Reddening Lepiota *(Lepiota Americana)* and the Shaggy Parasol *(Lepiota/Chlorophyllum rachodes).*

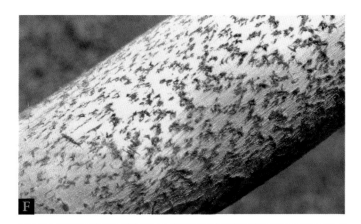

⚜ **Figure F:** Here is an example of the brown scales on the stem of the *Macrolepiota procera* that somewhat resemble herringbone.

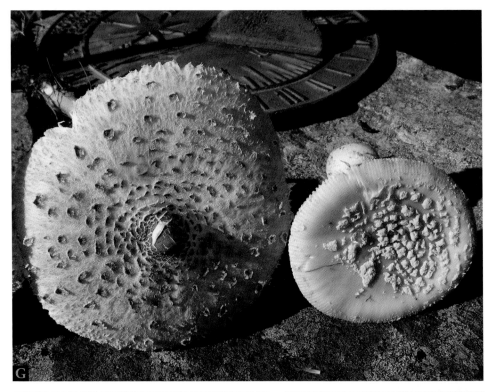

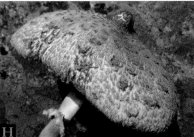

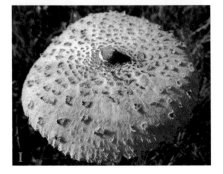

❧**Figure G:** The Parasol Mushroom is on the left and an *Amanita* on the right. You must take care to avoid the *Amanita*. Parasols have attached regular patterned brown scales on the cap, a central knob, and a patterned stem. They are not any shade of yellow. The stem will be enlarged at the base but not growing from a cup as an *Amanita* does. Other differences are the *Amanita* has irregular patches rather than scales, radial lines at the cap margin, no central knob, a hanging or mostly absent veil, and a bulbous stem usually growing from a cup or sac. ❧**Figure H:** A browner specimen of the Parasol Mushroom ❧**Figure I:** Top view shows the scales and central protrusion of *Macrolepiota procera*.

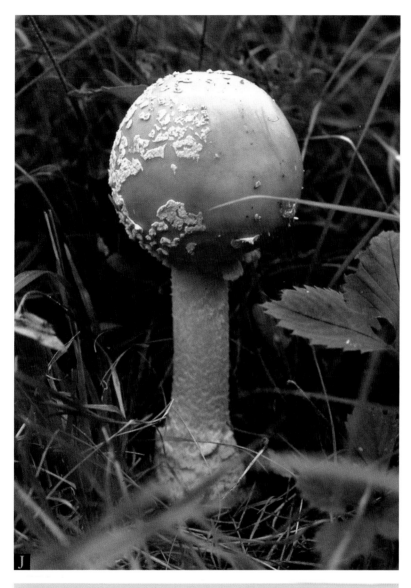

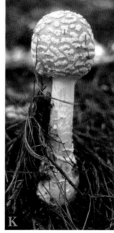

🌿**Figure J:** This is not a Parasol Mushroom—it is an *Amanita* and should never be eaten because it is poisonous. Note that the cap has irregular patches rather than scales. 🌿**Figure K:** This is not a Parasol Mushroom—it is an example of a poisonous *Amanita*. Any similar mushroom with white patches or a hanging veil or radial lines at the cap margin should always be avoided.

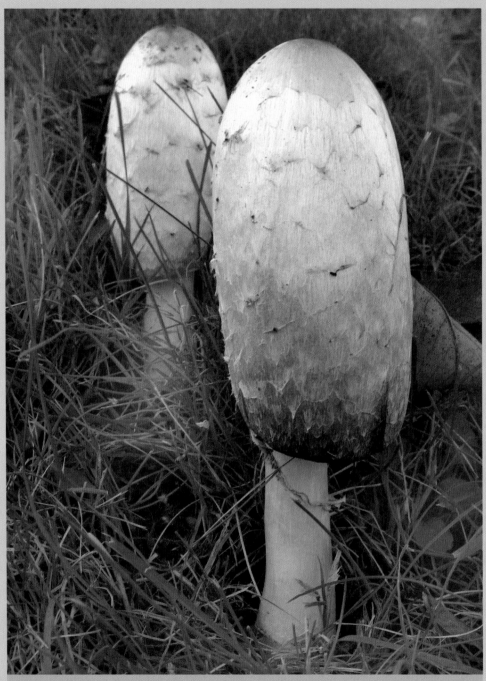

Shaggy Mane *(Coprinus comatus)*.

Chapter Eight

Shaggy Mane
(Coprinus comatus)

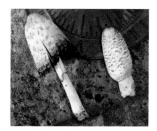

Shaggy Mane
(Coprinus comatus).

The Shaggy Mane, also occasionally called the Lawyers Wig, is a distinctive and easy to recognize mushroom. Its size, shape, and tendency to grow in tight groups make it easy to spot even from considerable distance. The *Coprinus comatus* has an elongated bullet-shaped, shaggy cap, with brownish upturned scales and a straight, fairly smooth stem.

Cap (pileus): The cap is shaggy, scaly, whitish, one to two inches wide, two to six inches tall, and it becomes inky and goocy as it expands eventually leaving just the stem. Scales are upturned and whitish tan to reddish brown.

Gills (lamellae): The Shaggy Mane has white, close, free gills that eventually become black and inky.

Stem (stipe): The stem is fibrous, hollow, straight, and white to tannish in color with a partial veil on the lower to middle area. The stem usually tapers somewhat, becoming slightly thinner near the top.

Flesh: The *Coprinus comatus* has white, quite soft, and easily broken flesh.

Spores: The Shaggy Mane makes black spore prints.

When and where to find them (ecology): The Shaggy Mane grows in summer and fall in grass, wood chips, rocky, or hard-packed soil and often appears shortly after a soaking rain. This species may grow singly or scattered but often in large, tightly packed groups. Some years they are quite common in city and suburban locations, pastures, lawns, gardens, along driveways, and so forth. Sometimes *Coprinus comatus* are found in huge quantities, presenting quite a dilemma because they require almost immediate preparation.

Preparation: Specimens should be collected at an early stage before they become inky. Because they will also turn inky within a few hours of picking, you should prepare them almost immediately. The refrigerator will slow down the process somewhat, but this species will not keep. The Shaggy Mane has a pleasant, subtle flavor that is quite mild so you may lose their flavor if you mix them with strong-flavored foods or other mushrooms. The *Coprinus comatus* are best sautéed, deep-fried in tempura, and served as a stand-alone dish. I do not think they can be dried. Grilling or pickling may be a possibility. This species will be satisfactory with eggs, cheese, white sauces, milder vegetables, chicken, fish, and other foods you associate with white wines.

Comments: Although the Shaggy Mane is quite easy to identify, I hesitated to add them because of their very short window of usability and their passing resemblance to *Coprinus atramentarius,* which can cause trouble when consumed with alcohol. Quite common some years, the Shaggy Mane has a nice but light flavor.

The *Coprinus comatus* can be used for dyeing wool, some fabrics, and paper. This species will yield a gray-green color with wool when ammonia is used as a mordant and a bayberry color when cooked in an iron pot.

You may have luck making a slurry for propagating Shaggy Manes in your lawn: Placing your older inky caps in water for a day or so to capture the spores in solution. Then pour the water on your lawn. You might also throw the caps on your lawn or wood chips.

Figure A: This *Coprinus atramentarius* has a smooth cap. Although considered edible by some, consuming alcohol with your meal will make you quite ill. One can have a problem if they drink alcohol a day or two later. **Figure B:** A Shaggy Mane *(Coprinus comatus)* at a perfect stage for harvest. **Figure C:** This Shaggy Mane is becoming very inky. **Figure D:** *Coprinus atramentarius* will turn into black, inky goop in a day or two.

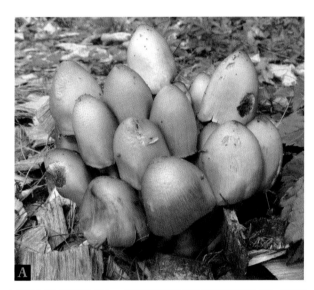

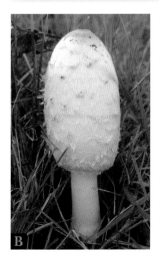

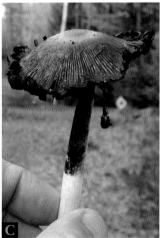

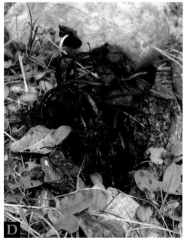

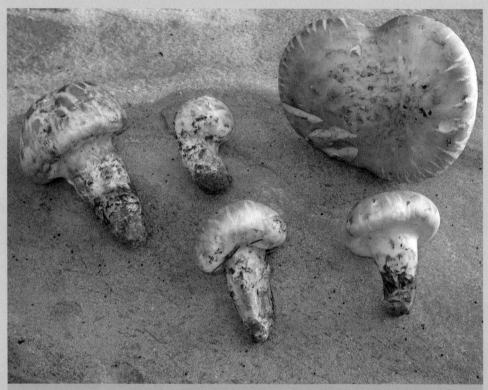
Matsutake at different growth stages.

Chapter Nine

Matsutake
(Tricholoma magnivelare)

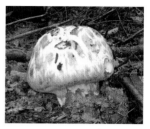

Recently emerged
Matsutake showing
reddish brown
scales.

September brings Matsutake season (pronounced maht-SOO-tah-keh). Somehow word of the cash value of this species has spread. Because they wholesale for six- to ten-dollars a pound, depending on grade, finding as few as ten to fifteen pounds in a morning is an profitable adventure. The folks who collect this species are extremely secretive about their stands and their methods of finding them. I once met some people who had found more than fifty pounds one Sunday morning and were leaving a broker's with some very decent checks.

Matsutake is an important ceremonial mushroom in Japan, often given in wooden presentation boxes to celebrate autumn. Popular as a corporate gift, it is a great honor to receive a pair of Matsutake with a pair of sake glasses. Matsutake commands astounding prices in Japan. Tightly closed caps, untrimmed stems, and moderate sizes in the four- to seven-inch range are preferred. Matsutake collected for the Japan market should never be trimmed.

Cap (pileus): The cap measures from two to more than eight inches across. It is convex at first, becoming flat. The cap is white as it first emerges from the duff and becomes tannish with reddish brown scales. It smells like dirty socks with a hint of cinnamon.

Gills (lamellae): The gills of the *Tricholoma magnivelare* are close and attached, and they are whitish, becoming a bit tan with age. The gills stain pinkish brown when bruised.

Stem (stipe): The stem ranges between two to six inches tall and three-fourths of an inch to two inches wide. Whitish in color, the stem has a white veil, which breaks irregularly; and the stem develops reddish brown scales but remains white above the soft ring. It often reaches deep into the soil or duff and can be swollen near the base then coming almost to a point.

Flesh: The flesh is white and firm.

Spores: The spore print of the Matsutake is white.

When and where to find them (ecology): Matsutake form a mycorrhizal relationship with trees. Although Matsutake are called the Pine Mushroom, they tend to grow under hemlock in this part of the country. This species comes in September and October around central Maine. Alternating cold nights and warm days seem to stimulate fruit growth. Some people have suggested that I look under red pine; however, I have checked the red pine on my own property and some other large, planted stands without finding any Matsutake. In fact, I have never found much of any type of mushroom under red pine except False Morels. I have found Matsutake under spruce. However, stands of older hemlocks around lakes and woodland streams are the most likely location for large stands of Matsutake. They may be found under Pitch Pine on Cape Cod.

During the entire season in 2006, I found only five Matsutake. Most collectors said 2006 was an off year, but at the broker's some hunters brought in quite a few. I was, however, successful at finding the stands of other specimens that had already been picked. In one case, a person had tied black thread to a tree branch at the edge of the road stringing it into the woods a considerable distance to his or her patch of Matsutake. I could still see the holes left behind.

In order to be successful at finding Matsutake, you should look for humps in the duff where specimens are popping up but not yet showing. If you find one, there could be several others under the same tree. These are likely to be the best ones with caps still unopened. Matsutake may only pop out of the ground slightly even when mature. But once you see the caps above the duff, they have often passed the point of being "A grade." The stem can be fairly deep in the ground so you may want to push your fingers into the dirt to pull up the entire fruit body because Matsutake are not sellable with trimmed stems. Be gentle in the soil and cover your holes with duff. If any mycelium comes out with the stem put it back in the hole. Although some people use a rake to find the emerging buttons, this practice may cause serious or irreparable damage to the habitat.

Preparation: Matsutake have quite an assertive flavor that you may need to get used to, and the smell can be off putting. With their unusual spicy taste, Matsutake are good sautéed or tempura-fried. With cooking, the off smell dissipates. The Japanese use Matsutake prepared with rice, in soups, as well as grilled and then eaten with a sauce made with soy sauce and vinegar.

Comments: I have yet to find more than a few Matsutake in a season. It is a busy time of year for many mushrooms, though, so I do not always put in a lot of time looking for this species specifically. The Matsutake is more of something I find when hunting in a general way or looking for King Boletes.

The kind folks at the local mushroom brokers have been giving me some of their Matsutake throwaways. I have tried spreading and burying the fruit bodies under hemlocks and red pines on my property, hoping to start a crop.

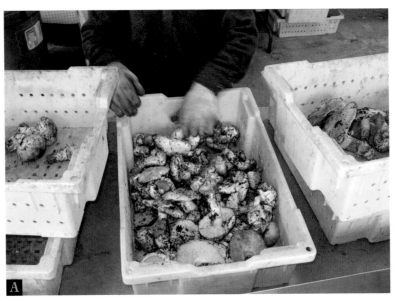

A

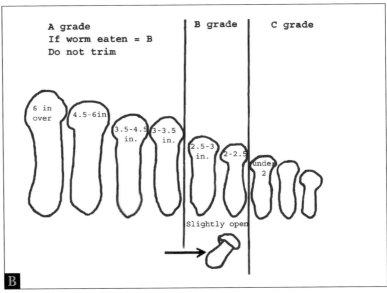

A grade
If worm eaten = B
Do not trim

B grade

C grade

6 in over

4.5-6in

3.5-4.5 in.

3-3.5 in.

2.5-3 in.

2-2.5

under 2

Slightly open

B

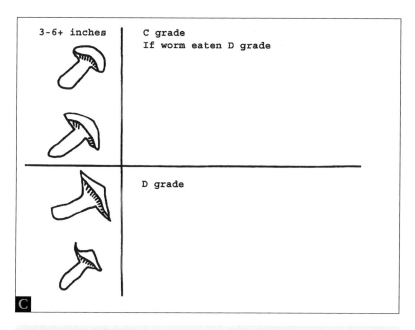

Figure A: These Matsutake are being graded for the Japanese market. Figure B: Sample of a Matsutake grading chart for Grade A, B, and C. Figure C: Matsutake grading chart for Grade C and D. Figure D: Matsutake grading chart for Grade D and E.

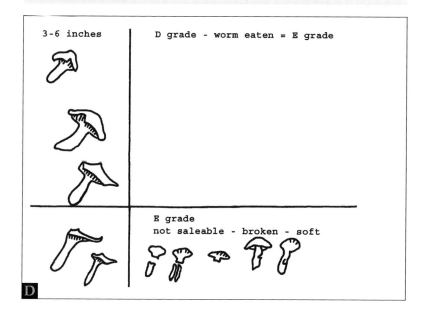

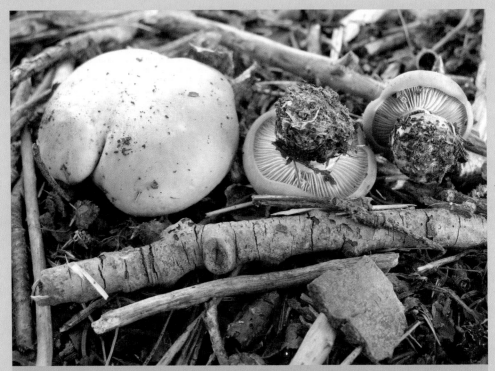

Young, shaded Blewits have pronounced blue or lavender coloring.

Chapter Ten

Blewit

(Lepista nuda)

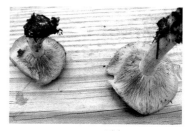

Older specimens of *Lepista nuda* can develop elongated stems and tanner color. Hints of color persist in the gills.

When the Maitake and King Bolete season starts to fade in Maine, it can seem like mushroom season is over. However, if you continue to search around oaks and edges, you are likely to spot Blewits. A very distinctive-tasting mushroom, whose flavor is hard to describe, I hesitate to call it bitter, though the taste may have a slightly bitter edge. It has a spicy, fairly strong flavor that can only be described as Blewit-flavored.

Cap (pileus): The cap ranges from one to six inches wide, is bluish lavender in color, convex with inrolled edges when young—with a shape somewhat similar to a button mushroom. As the Blewit matures, the cap becomes broadly convex, often developing an upturned, wavy edge and tends to fade toward tan with age. Blewits seem to maintain their color better in shadier locations and have a fragrant aroma.

Gills: The gills are lavender, fading toward tan-brown with age; are close together, and have a notched attachment to the stem.

Stem (stipe): The stem of a young specimen is likely to be thick, enlarged at the base, and one inch or less in length. As it ages, the stem can stretch out to several inches and fades toward tan. Mycelium is attached to the stem at the base and will have a slight bluish lavender tint.

Flesh: The *Lepista nuda* has whitish lavender flesh.

Spores: Whitish buff with possibly a slightly pinkish tint.

When and where to find them (ecology): Blewits start to grow when nights start getting cold and approach frost temperatures, which in this area usually occurs in mid- to late October or slightly later. The species can continue appearing until December if the weather stays somewhat mild. Moderate December temperatures are more likely in coastal areas.

Places with compost, such as grass clippings, wood chips, and wood waste from raking, seem to be the most suitable habitats. Natural compost created on the ground around oaks and other hardwoods also supports Blewits. Check the edges of parks and cemeteries where the landscapers dump this type of refuse as well as areas where lawns border woods and bushes.

This species can be harder to identify if specimens are older because of the tan-brown color and stretched-out profile they develop. As with many species, every once in a while a really huge specimen will appear which can be confusing. For example, I once saw some Blewits growing inside a local greenhouse that had faded to tan-brown and one of them was nine inches across. I consulted other knowledgeable collectors online to verify my identification. I discovered that the gills will still maintain a slight hint of color.

Preparation: Be sure to cook Blewits thoroughly because they are mildly toxic when raw. Some people have sensitivity to this species so sample a very small amount the first time. Blewits are well matched with white wine and foods associated with white wine. The Blewit's unique, assertive flavor enhances dishes of veal, pork, fish, poultry, cheese, rice, and pasta.

I strongly recommend that you first sample Blewits either sautéed or by another simple process that showcases their unique flavor so that you can appreciate that flavor before you try preparing them in a more complex dish. I have enjoyed them immensely sautéed, deep-fried in tempura batter, and microwaved. Whether deep lavender or tan in color, Blewits seem to become similar in color in the frying pan with a slight lavender tint. I have not yet found enough specimens to dry them.

Comments: There are other species of mushrooms that are lavender or purple so you need to be careful when identifying Blewits. For example, the species from the *Cortinarius* genus, which you should *always* avoid, have a cobwebby veil, most often a bulbous base, and rust-colored spores. You should also

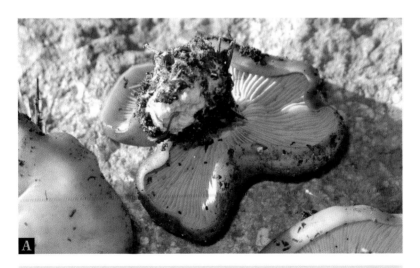

Figure A: Compare the colors of the specimen in the center with the two located in the lower corners to see how coloration can vary.

avoid species of *Entolomas,* which are likely to have thinner stems and pink spores. Be sure to make a spore print.

Beginning collectors should avoid all mushrooms with pink or rust color spores. Unless you are absolutely sure that you have harvested Blewits, do not attempt to taste them.

Blewits are relatively easy to propagate: Put a clean fruit body into a jar filled with unsterilized, fresh, clean, dampened hardwood sawdust. Once the mycelium begins to show signs of growth, pull the mushroom out so it does not fester. When the mycelium has grown through all of the sawdust, it can be broken up and planted outdoors into shady locations with composting soil.

Blewits can be used for dyeing textiles, paper, and wool. When cooked in an iron pot with ammonia as a mordant, Blewits will yield a grass-green color.

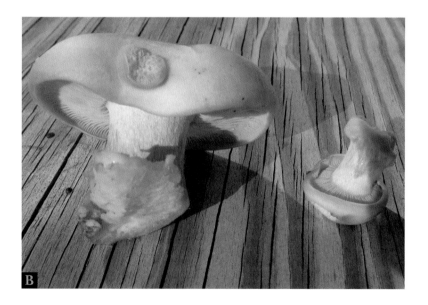

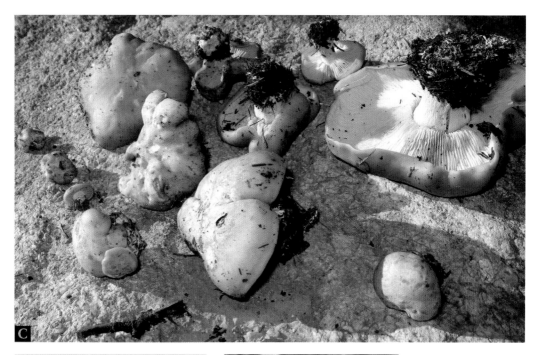

C

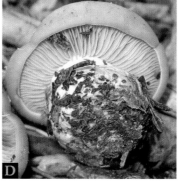

D

Figure B: These light colored specimens were heavily shaded. **Figure C:** Different sizes, shapes, and coloration from the same stand. **Figure D:** A very young specimen. **Figure E:** This is an older tannish brown *Lepista nuda*. **Figure F:** A close-up view of the notched gill attachment.

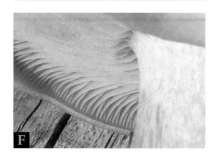

F

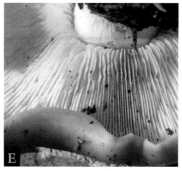

E

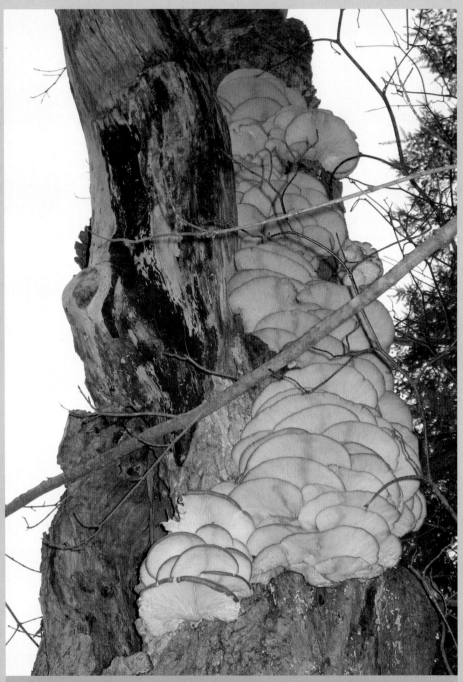

Pleurotus ostreatus on a dying sugar maple.

Chapter Eleven

Oyster Mushrooms

(Pleurotus ostreatus, P. populinus, and Others)

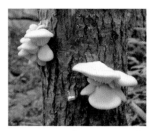

Pleurotus populinus on a dead poplar/aspen log.

I n central Maine, two species of "true" Oyster Mushrooms are predominate: *Pleurotus ostreatus* and *P. populinus.* The taxonomy of the species of *Pleurotus* is still in flux. These are more of a complex. *Pleurotus ostreatus* grows in the fall to early winter. The almost identical *P. populinus,* a recently described species, grows in late spring and occasionally throughout the season exclusively on poplar/aspen trees. Before *P. populinus* was defined as a distinct species, it was considered a spring variant of *P. ostreatus* with a white spore print. The Oyster Mushroom previously known as *Pleurotus sapidus* is known as the "true" *P. ostreatus.* It generally has a lavender-lilac spore print if allowed to develop any thickness. These species are good edibles with medicinal properties.

Cap (pileus): The cap of *Pleurotus ostreatus* and *P. populinus* measures one to twelve inches wide and one-half to one and one-half inches thick. The cap is convex and semicircular to fan-shaped, overlapping in large bunches. Both species of Oyster Mushrooms usually have a strong aniselike aroma. Older fruit bodies may develop an unpleasant smell. The color of the cap of *P. ostreatus* is likely to be tan to brown but can be whitish, grayish, or even gray-blue. The gray-blue color, though, is more likely to be seen in cultivated *P. ostreatus* of European origin. *P. populinus* has a whitish ivory cap.

Gills (lamellae): The gills of both species are fairly close together running down the stem and are white, light gray, or tannish in color. *Pleurotus populinus* is likely to be whitish ivory, whereas *P. ostreatus* will have more variation in color—usually tan to brown.

Stem (stipe): The stem of either species is usually nonexistent to stubby unless the specimen is growing on top of a log and bunched together (cespitose).

Flesh: Both *Pleurotus ostreatus* and *P. populinus* have thick, white, and nonbruising flesh.

Spores: The *Pleurotus ostreatus* makes a whitish gray or lavender-lilac spore print. The thicker the spore print is, the more likely some color will show. *P. populinus* makes a white to very slightly grayish spore print.

When and where to find them (ecology): The *Pleurotus populinus* is mostly found in late May and early June on dead poplar/aspen species exclusively. I find them on both quaking aspen and eastern cottonwood. The trees are likely to be between six and thirty feet tall with few or no branches. *P. populinus* may appear sporadically throughout the summer especially after a heavy rain. I have not found them on a living tree, but it is possible. They have a strongly anise-almond aroma.

The *Pleurotus ostreatus* is found from middle of fall to mid-December and seems to prefer sugar maple and occasionally beech or other hardwoods. *P. ostreatus* are likely to be on living mature trees, with obvious signs the trees are dying, or

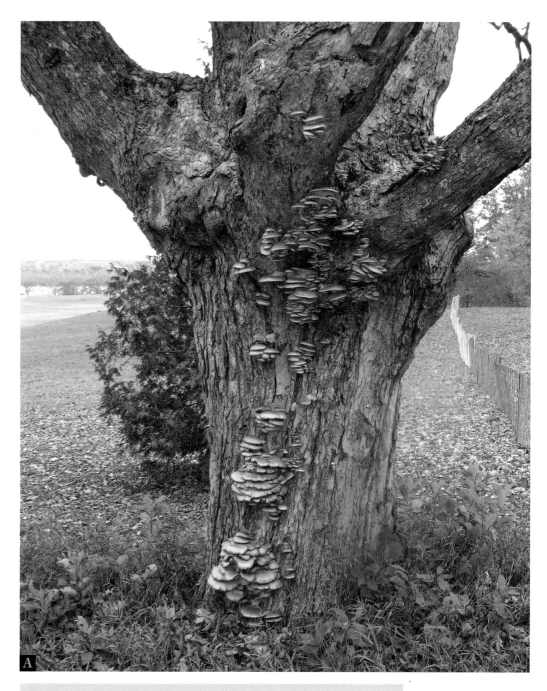

❧ **Figure A:** *Pleurotus ostreatus* on sugar maple.

occasionally on dead wood. This species of Oyster Mushroom can grow very high in the tree and in enormous numbers. I have noted they often grow on sugar maples that have been tapped for sap in the spring, which suggests that the creation of holes for the spiles may allow for entry of spores. Noting the locations of sugaring operations in the spring should help you find them in the fall. *P. ostreatus* also has a strongly anise-almond aroma. They can be found year round in the produce section of most supermarkets. You may be able to collect spores from the supermarket mushrooms for study or propagation.

Preparation: Both *Pleurotus ostreatus* and *P. populinus* are fairly tasty when sautéed, though the flavor is a bit understated and the texture can be a bit chewy. When cooked with tempura batter, their goodness really comes out. Although both species have an enjoyable anise-almond aroma when first picked, the aroma often dissipates within a few hours. However, if you pick and cook them within a short time, the tempura will retain some of the anise-almond character. Neither species is very successful as a dried product because the texture is leathery when reconstituted. Additionally, as a powder, the flavor is far less exciting than many other mushroom powders. In fact, I consider both species to be a bit overrated as an edible. They can easily become chewy by a number of techniques. However, I have found that they make a satisfactory duxelles. These species should remain popular, because they are easy to grow, possess medicinal properties, and are quite common.

Comments: *Pleurotus ostreatus* or *P. populinus* look exactly alike except for slight color differences. Either one left sitting on a sheet of glass will eventually drop an enormous amount of spores in a wide circle. Spores are then easy to collect by scraping them of with a razor blade. The spores may be somewhat sticky but this seems to be okay. You can also place your less-than-excellent caps in a bucket of water, which will infuse the water with billions of spores to make a slurry. Then pour the slurry onto injured trees, logs, or wood chips.

Mycelium of *Pleurotus ostreatus* or *P. populinus* grown in the same petri dish do not mate with each other, which indicates that they are separate species. *P. ostreatus* is quite easy to cultivate growing on a wide variety of substrates, whereas *P. populinus* seems to like only poplar/aspen trees.

Using spores, I could not get vigorous mycelium to grow on potato agar. Cutting off the stems and bark from *P. ostreatus* and placing them in wet sawdust or soaked dowels plugs will often result in aggressive growth, creating spawn you can use for stump, log, or other inoculation purposes.

I have a few dozen *P. populinus* logs in my yard, which I have brought from the woods. I cut them into three-foot bolts with my chainsaw and stack them in the shade near my house—a strategy you may want to try for growing wild mushrooms in your yard. When found in the woods, after a heavy fruiting, the wood becomes softer and insects move in. This attracts the hairy and pileated woodpeckers that often dismantle the tree, leaving just a pile of chips on the ground. However, woodpeckers do not bother the logs too much that I have laid out in my yard.

Species of *Pleurotus* have some medicinal value and therefore should probably remain on your menu. There have been some studies that indicate that polysaccharides in *P. ostreatus* may be useful in the treatment of prostate cancer and other cancers.

Noted mycologist Paul Stamets has demonstrated that strains of Oyster Mushrooms he has developed can effectively perform bioremediation by breaking down the structure of

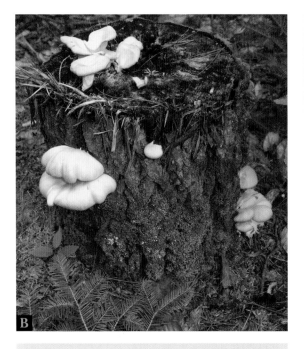

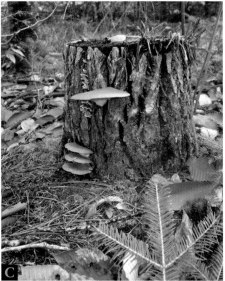

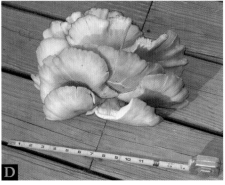

❧ **Figure B:** Taken in October 2007, this image shows *Pleurotus populinus* growing from a poplar stump that I had inoculated with *Pleurotus ostreatus* two years earlier. These had the typical whitish ivory color and white spores. ❧ **Figure C:** The *Pleurotus ostreatus* mentioned in Figure B showed up on the same poplar stump six weeks later. These specimens had a slightly lavender spore print. These, from spawn I ordered from www.fungi.com, have a slightly different look than the native variety being browner, flatter, and somewhat thinner. Two varieties of Oyster Mushrooms growing on one stump. This is the first positive result from many stump inoculations. Turkey Tails are also sharing this stump. ❧ **Figure D:** *Pleurotus ostreatus* caps measuring eight to ten inches wide. ❧ **Figure E:** *Pleurotus populinus*. ❧ **Figure F:** *Pleurotus ostreatus* on sugar maple.

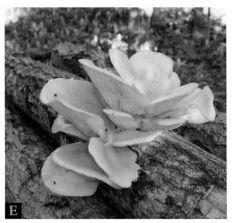

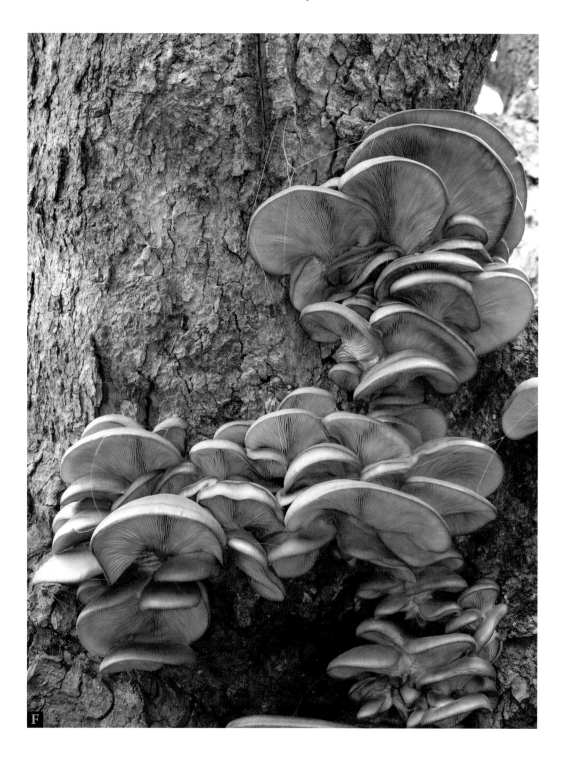

hydrocarbon molecules of diesel fuel, oil, gasoline, PCBs, and similar pollutants. There are many bioremediation strategies possible using species of *Pleurotus*. I have experimented with growing Oyster Mushroom mycelium on a number of unusual substances. I successfully grew a few mushrooms on an old cotton shirt and have grown mycelium on dryer lint and coffee grounds.

Oyster Mushrooms can be used for dyeing wool, some fabrics, and paper. When using an iron pot and ammonia as modifiers, the species will yield a gray-green color with wool.

Pleurotus pulmonarius grows in summer and is somewhat uncommon in Maine. It usually has a stem and often will be found on conifers or oak. It is edible and good. Also found occasionally in summer, *Pleurotus dryinus,* has a feltlike stem that tends to join off center under the cap. *P. dryinus,* which is edible, grows singly or in smaller numbers on hardwoods, such as maple.

Hypsizygus species are a taxonomic problem, and there is conflicting information in field guides and on Web sites. *Hypsizygus tessulatus,* often known as an Elm Oyster, may be found on various hardwoods in fall. *H. tessulatus* has a prominent stem and gills that do not run down the stem. *H. tessulatus* is edible.

When compared to species of *Pleurotus,* the Late Fall Oyster *(Panellis serotinus)* is brownish with green and yellow tones and has slightly different gills that have a sharp ending at the stem. Because the *Panellis serotinus* is quite chewy and often slightly bitter, they may be a culinary disappointment.

Angel Wings *(Pleurocybella porrigens)* are thin, white, and grow on conifers. There have been some reports of poisoning recently although most field guides list them as edible. Therefore, the safest course is to avoid Angel Wings.

Species of *Crepidotus* are very small and have a brown spore print. They should not be eaten.

Lentinus/Lentinellus are tough and they have hairy brown caps, an off smell, and a bad taste. Remember, young and fresh Oyster Mushrooms have a lovely aroma!

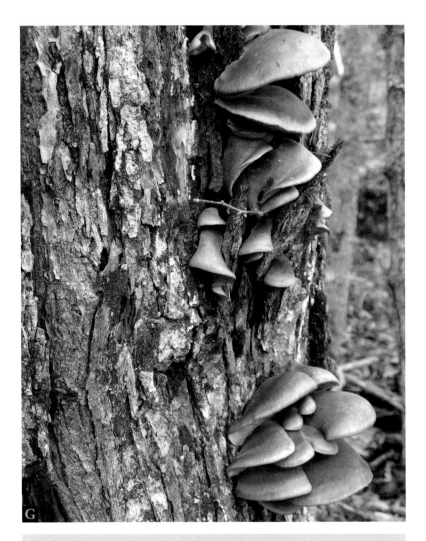

Figure G: The Late Fall Oyster *(Panellus serotinus),* being fairly tough and often bitter, is edible but not as tasty as Pleurotus species.

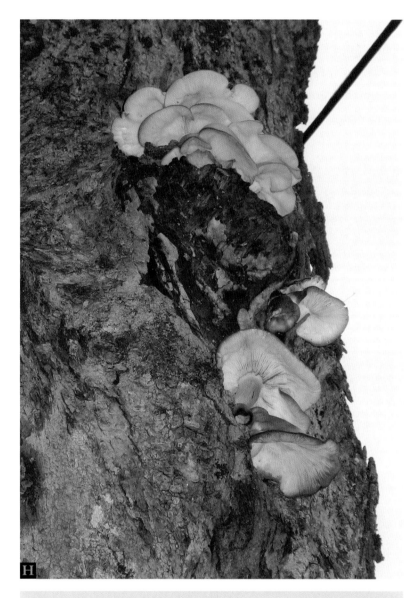

Figure H: *Hypsizgus tessulatus* on sugar maple. Figure I: *Hypsizgus tessulatus*. Figure J: *Pleurotus dryinus* in midsummer on maple. Figure K: *Hypsizgus tessulatus*. Figure L: Orange Mock Oyster (*Phyllotopsis nidulans*), on dead poplar, is too bitter and tough to eat. Figure M: The Late Fall Oyster often has some yellowish and/or greenish tones.

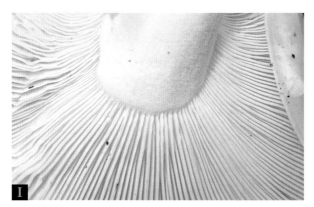

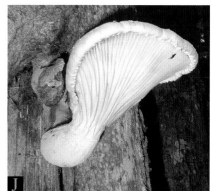

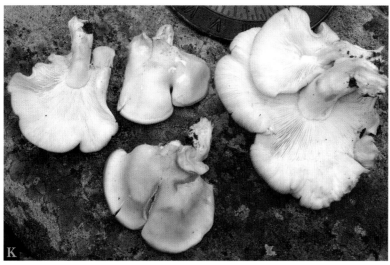

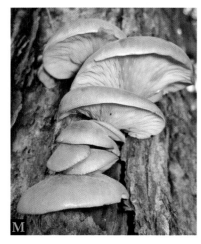

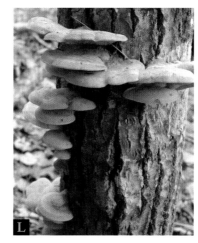

Section Three

Mushrooms with Pores

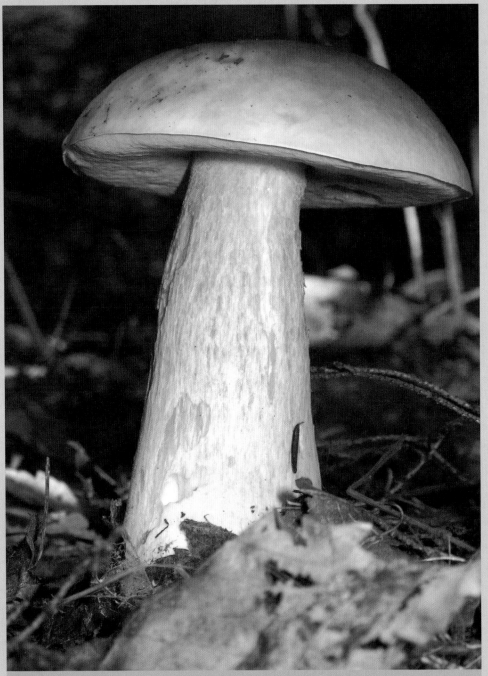

This specimen is typical for this region.

Chapter Twelve

King Bolete

(Boletus edulis and Others*)*

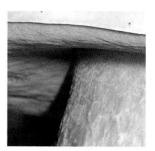

The reticulation at the top of the stem is very fine in this specimen.

The King Bolete is a very popular, delicious, meaty mushroom that grows throughout the world. A few of its many names are Cep, Porcini, *Steinpilz,* and Penny Bun. It is a complex of closely related species with similar looks, habitat, and flavor wherever it is found. Highly variable in coloration and a favorite and familiar mushroom that has been drawn, painted, and sculpted by artists, the King Bolete is often very large and stately with a thick club-shaped stem, thick cap, and an impressive "kingly" appearance.

Cap (pileus): Ranging from two to more than ten inches wide, the cap is smooth, quite thick, and a bit sticky in damp weather. The cap is convex, becoming flat at maturity. The color of the cap varies from light brown to reddish brown. It is dense when young and becomes spongy with age. The aroma is pleasant.

Tubes (hymenophore): The tubes of the King Bolete are sunken around the stalk. The pores are closely spaced, small, and quite hard when young and white, changing to yellowish then to pea-soup green to greenish brown and becoming fairly soft.

Stem (stipe): The King Bolete stem is very thick and club-shaped. When young, the stem is often almost as thick at the bottom as the cap is wide. The stem is usually finely reticulated, meaning it has a net-shaped raised pattern on its surface. The reticulation is whitish and most pronounced near the top. The color of the stem can vary from whitish cream to reddish brown. It can become cylindrical at maturity.

Flesh: The flesh is white and dense in younger specimens and becomes softer at maturity. Generally nonstaining, the flesh has a pleasant flavor when tasted raw.

Spores: The spore print is olive brown.

When and where to find them (ecology): Mycorrhizal, King Boletes are most often found under oak and hemlock trees especially where sphagnum mosses are present and fairly common under most varieties of spruce. I have also seen them with birch, beech, apple, mixed woods and found *Boletus pinophilus* with eastern white pine. I should note that the fruit bodies I have collected under white pines were very similar to *B. edulis* and fruited in the fall. In Maine *B. edulis* will be usually be found from the end of August through the middle November; and occasionally, they will appear earlier. Some field guides say *B. edulis* are uncommon in the East, which is not remotely true in my experience. Although the last three years have been quite poor, usually *B. edulis* are quite abundant. In 2002 I found almost enough specimens to pay my tuition for the two college courses I was taking. I actually collected ninety pounds from one location and more than forty pounds at another. Indeed, I found so many that year that I had to sell most of them.

In June and July you may find the very similar-looking *Boletus variipes* under oak, which has a tan, dry cap and usually a more strongly reticulated and cylindrical stem. Its flavor is not quite as sublime as the King Bolete, and some *B. variipes* I have found had a slightly bitter edge. It is available at a time when there is not much else to find. *Xanthoconium separans* has yellow pores and usually lilac hues on the stem. Spotted bolete *(X. affine)* has white to yellow pores and a reddish brown cap often with yellow spots. Both are good edibles. The Bitter Bolete *(Tylopilus felleus)* has a dark web on the stalk and a very bitter taste.

Preparation: King Boletes are excellent sautéed and even microwaved. The flesh of young specimens is crunchy with a somewhat nutty flavor, but the flesh of older specimens may become quite soft. *Boletus edulis* occasionally have a slightly bitter edge. For the pan, you may want to remove the pore layer on older specimens; however, for drying, you can leave them on. *B. edulis* is outstanding dried and reconstituted. The drying concentrates its flavor and ameliorates any slight bitterness. When powdered, they impart strong flavor that is great for soup, gravy, meat loaf, pasta, sauce, and so forth. But do not use too much powder because it can become too strong.

Comments: Early finds of *Boletus edulis* may be infested with fly larvae so be sure to check the bottom of the stem for holes. Once cold weather sets in, this becomes less of a problem. This species often comes up most strongly around the time of frost. Frost or near-frost conditions reduce infestation problems greatly. Sometimes *B. edulis* can be gargantuan. In 1999 I found actually one with a fourteen-inch cap that was more than four inches thick. The stem was close to four inches thick, as well. This King Bolete weighed more than two pounds.

In summer and early fall, you may find *Tylopilus felleus,* the Bitter Bolete. Usually tan or reddish tan with a similar colored stem, the species has fairly prominent reticulation. Its pores often have a pinkish tinge. It is very similar to *Boletus edulis* in appearance but the *Tylopilus felleus* has a truly unpalatable level of bitterness. Early in the season, it is best to sample a very small bit of flesh from your finds. You will spit out *T. felleus* immediately.

Boletus edulis can be used for dyeing textiles, paper, and wool. When ammonia is used as a mordant, this species will yield a chrome yellow color.

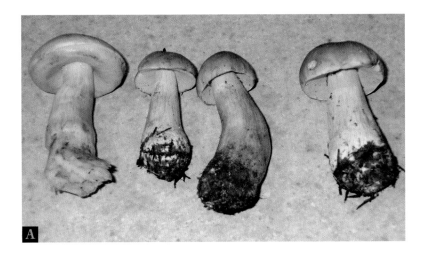

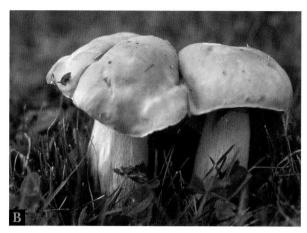

❧ **Figure A:** Young early season *Boletus edulis.* ❧ **Figure B:** Choice-looking, fairly large *Boletus edulis.* ❧ **Figure C:** *Boletus variipes.* ❧ **Figure D:** The pores have become brownish and overmature on the larger specimen. Pores can be removed quite easily.

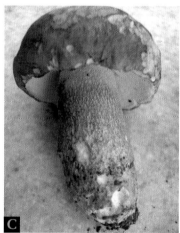

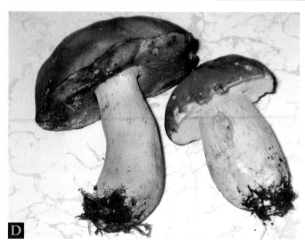

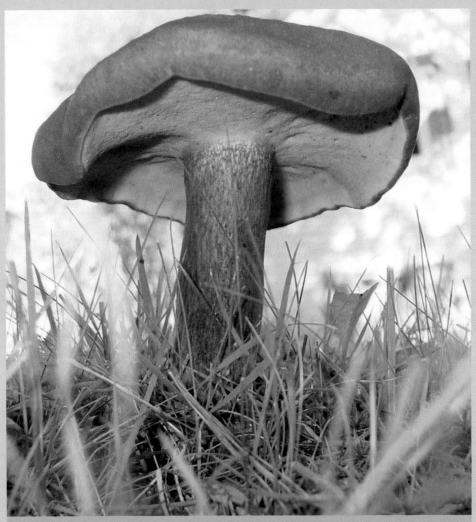

A mature specimen showing the yellow pores.

Chapter Thirteen

Two-Colored Bolete
(Boletus bicolor)

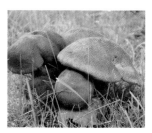

A cluster of
Boletus bicolor.

Cap (pileus): The cap of the Two-colored Bolete ranges from two to six inches wide and from pinkish to dark red, often with some yellow tones near the margin. When young, the cap is convex, smooth, and dry with a somewhat velvety surface; as it matures, the cap flattens, often cracks, and changes to yellow-brown in color. In rare cases the cap can be yellow.

Tubes (hymenophore): The tubes may be sunken around the stalk when first opening but tend to descend the stalk as the cap opens wider. The minute, angular pores are yellow slowly bruising dark blue. The blue bruising can tend to lighten after a few minutes.

Stem (stipe): The pink or red stem can be quite thick and club-shaped, and occasionally it splits as shown in Figures A, B, and D. The stem can thin a bit and become more cylindrical as it grows with yellow tones mostly near the top.

Flesh: The flesh is strongly yellow, then slowly bruises to blue.

Spores: The Two-colored Bolete makes a brown spore print.

When and where to find them (ecology): I have found specimens between a Norway maple and a yew. The *Boletus bicolor* can grow in profusion, often coming up in several flushes from late June to mid-September. Mycorrhizal, the Two-colored Bolete often associates with oak and other hardwoods and usually grows separately or in small clusters. Occasionally, the *B. bicolor* will grow in large groups, with overlapping caps.

Preparation: This species is truly an excellent edible, ranking at least as tasty as the King Bolete *(Boletus edulis)*. In addition to great flavor, specimens of the *B. bicolor* are visually appealing—real showstoppers—with their bright yellow, dense flesh that is edged in red. Younger dense specimens have a pleasant crunchy texture. Any slight bluishness tends to disappear during cooking. I have sautéed, grilled, and microwaved Two-colored Boletes with excellent results. I have also dried some; however, they do not have the pungent aroma of the King Bolete *(B. edulis)*.

Comments: The Two-colored Bolete is one of the best-tasting mushrooms you will find. Its unique flavor is not lost in complex dishes. Versatile to cook with, this species can be mixed with many types of foods, although you would likely want to avoid mixing them with more common mushrooms, such as the White Button/Cremini/Portobello Mushroom.

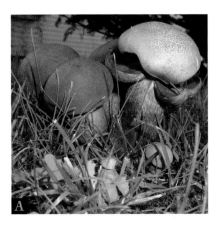 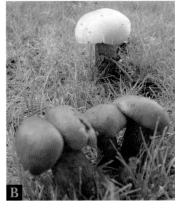

Boletes with red or orange pores should not be eaten. Beginners should also stay away from any deep blue-staining mushrooms. The Two-colored Bolete bears some resemblance to the poisonous *Boletus sensibilis,* which immediately bruises deep blue and is more brick to cinnamon color. *B. subvetipes* has orange or red pores, is also poisonous, and immediately bruises strongly blue to blue-black.

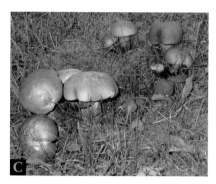 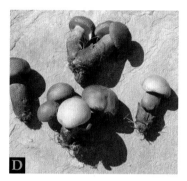

❧ **Figure A:** *Boletus bicolor* showing specimens with yellowish caps. ❧ **Figure B:** Atypical specimens of *Boletus bicolor.* ❧ **Figure C:** *Boletus bicolor* growing in a cluster and separately. ❧ **Figure D:** These Two-colored Boletes are typical of the way you may find them in small clusters and spread about. The yellow-capped specimens are not commonly found. ❧ **Figure E:** Two-colored Bolete shish kabob with Italian dressing marinade.

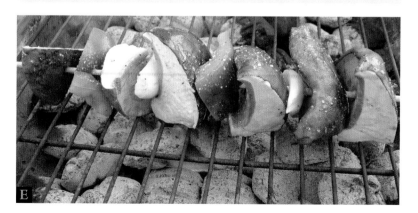

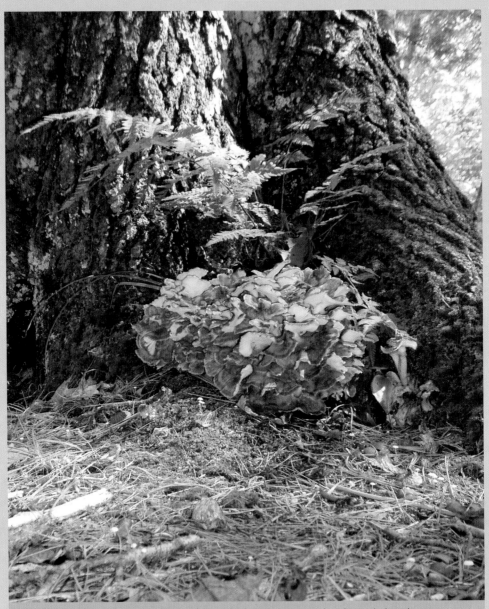

You will find ninety-eight percent of Maitake around oak and dead stumps.
Most years, I find them under a black locust.
Red maple is also a possible habitat.

Chapter Fourteen

Maitake

(Grifola frondosa)

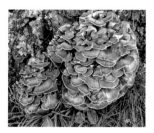

Look closely, there are actually two Maitake here.

Also known as Hen of the Woods, Ram's Head, Sheep's Head, and Cloud Mushroom, Maitake (pronounced my-TAH-keh) is the Japanese name for the edible fungus *Grifola frondosa*. I look forward to Labor Day when the Maitake begin to appear in Maine. Called the Dancing Mushroom probably because of the excitement generated by finding it, the Maitake has a distinctive smell and flavor. In addition to being a great edible, evidence is increasing that this species is highly medicinal, boosting the immune system to fight cancer and stabilizing blood sugar and blood pressure. The Maitake may also have antihypertensive and antidiabetic properties.

Fruit body: The *Grifola frondosa* is composed of clusters of flattened caps that can be similar to a feather duster or a sitting hen. The fruit body can measure from four to more than thirty-six inches across. From the bottom, the stem and branch structure may remind you of the underside of a cauliflower. The weight of the Maitake cluster usually ranges from three to fifteen pounds, but they can weigh much more. A local mushroom broker in Maine purchased an eighty-five pound specimen a few years back that required delivery on a child's plastic snow sled.

Cap (pileus): Each individual cap measures from three-fourths of an inch to more than three inches across, with grayish to brownish tones and often with a whitish zone in the middle of the cap. Caps are about one-eighth to one-fourth of an inch thick or even thinner.

Tubes (hymenophore): The tubes are very shallow, angular, and descend the stalk. The pore surface of the Maitake is grayish in younger specimens, becomes more white with age, and develops some yellow or brown tones as it passes its peak.

Stem (stipe): This species has a single central white stem with a complex branched structure that is similar to cauliflower or broccoli.

Flesh: The flesh is white and toughens a bit with age.

Spores: The Maitake makes a white spore print. The spores are fairly easy to propagate.

When and where to find them (ecology): The *Grifola frondosa* is found from the end of August until as late as early November in some years on mature oaks that often have dying branches. Look in parks; on lawns; along edges; and in low, somewhat wet areas. Red oak is a particularly likely host. Dead tree stumps should not be overlooked, either, considering that 2005 was an off year for Maitake and the only ones I found were by dead stumps. Ponds, lakes, and coastal areas with a lot of very mature oak are also likely places. A tree will often have several to many individual fruit bodies. I have found as many as thirteen around a single tree. They may grow all at once or sometimes come out over a period of two or three weeks. It is wise to keep checking a tree where you have already harvested some and to check the same locations for many years as they tend to reappear. Most years I find one or two under a specific black locust. One local mycologist even found one under a red maple this past season. Young and middle-aged healthy trees seldom harbor Maitake.

Preparation: For the table, Maitake may be the most versatile species of all. It has a unique, truly excellent flavor that neither overpowers nor is easily overpowered. Maitake is delicious sautéed, deep-fried, microwaved, boiled, and dried. It has an extremely pleasant, crunchy, very chewable texture all the way down the stem. I have heard that you can freeze them raw and break off pieces for cooking all winter. Sautéed Maitake freezes well, too.

If you find three or four *Grifola frondosa,* you can easily have twenty to fifty pounds of mushrooms, which is too much for immediate consumption. Maitake also makes excellent dux-elles (see Chapter Twenty-five). Drying is often necessary. Starting from the underside, pull at the individual caps and branches and they split right down to the bottom of the stem. They usually split thin enough to dry that way. Sometimes you need to split bottom pieces further. It is not very hard because the mushroom has a grain that the split follows. Try to keep the pieces less than one-fourth of an inch thick.

The flesh of the Maitake is edible all the way to the base of the stem. You may need to scrape bits of dirt or bark off of the cap surface and trim the cap edges. Dry the whole pieces at 110–120° in a dehydrator or low oven. The outer caps and branches that are thicker and a little tougher tend to take longer to dry. The thicker pieces can darken some and have less eye appeal so you may want to use them to make a powder for cooking. Leave the pieces that dry with nice, white, inner flesh and rehydrate them later. I occasionally use them dry as a cracker and eat them with cheese dip, hummus, and so forth.

Use the dried Maitake powder to add flavor to meat loaf, pasta sauce, gravy, béchamel-based sauces, and so on. Use the powder liberally because it has a subtle flavor. Maitake powder also makes a pleasant medicinal tea. I have also made a surprisingly pleasant Maitake-Reishi liquor.

Comments: This species has caused minor illness for at least a few people, although I have never met anyone who has had a problem with it. Maitake is often found in larger supermarkets. If you have health issues or take medication, there is a possibility of interaction. Check with your doctor. Many doctors are not well informed about mushrooms, though. As always, sample a small amount at first.

The Maitake vaguely resembles the much larger Berkeley's Polypore *(Bondarzewia berkeleyi)* and the Black-staining Polypore *(Meripilus giganteus),* both of which are nonpoisonous. I have tried Berkeley's Polypore and it is slightly bitter and just edible.

Maitake can be used for dyeing textiles, paper, and wool and will yield a soft yellow color when ammonia is used as a mordant. Because preparing this species for cooking or drying often leaves a lot of trimmed excess, dyeing may be a good use for it.

There is promising information being developed about the medicinal properties of Maitake. Unique beta-glucans are complex polysaccharides that enhance the function of the immune system. The American Cancer Society has positive things to say about this species, and there are breast cancer studies being conducted at Sloan-Kettering Cancer Center.

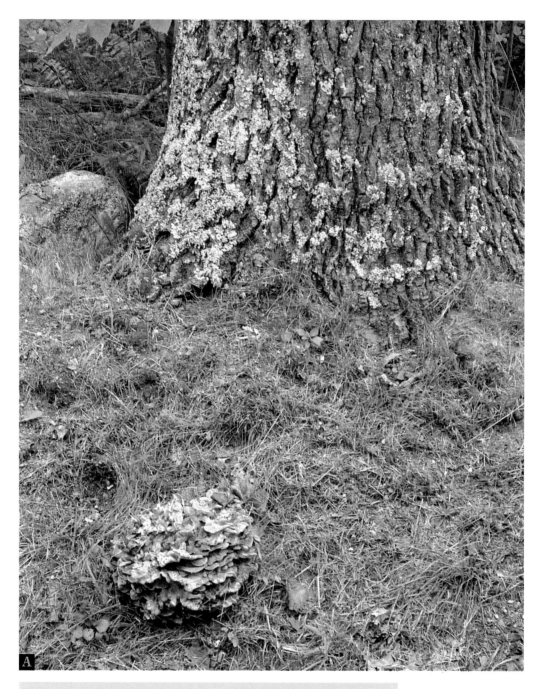

🌱 **Figure A:** Sometimes Maitake are located away from the stump.

On a personal note: In early 2004 I learned that my son had a sixth-grade classmate who was diagnosed with stage two malignant infiltrating brain cancer (astrocytoma). Located in the child's thalamus and around her hypothalamus / pituitary glands, the cancer was inoperable. She was given less than a year to live. Radiation and chemotherapy were not an option because of the location of the cancer. Further, the treatment would have prevented her from reaching puberty. She was on anticonvulsive medication only.

After hearing about this, I gave her mother about half a bushel of Maitake, which I had collected and dried. It was consumed as regular food at their house. Much to her doctor's surprise, the cancer stopped growing. Her tumor has not disappeared but it has not grown or progressed as doctors had expected it to. It has been four years with no new growth and the only medication is the anticonvulsive. She has reached puberty and is healthy and attending school regularly. Today, she has a boyfriend and is a typical tenth grader. She needs only six-month checkups at this point. The doctor stated that although this is not what she had expected, she is hopeful. I have continued to give the family a large bag of dried Maitake each fall.

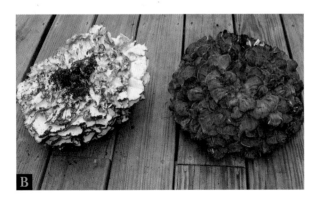

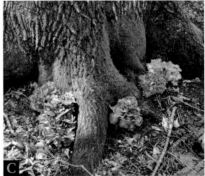

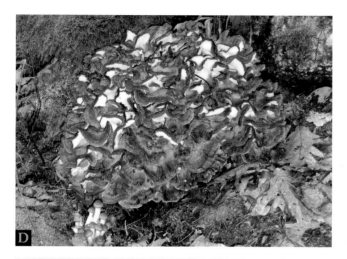

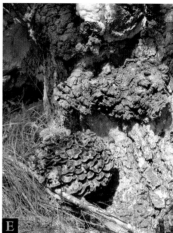

🌿 **Figure B:** Top (right) and underside (left) views of a *Grifola frondosa*. 🌿 **Figure C:** Here are five Maitake on one tree and four more are not shown. 🌿 **Figure D:** A choice-looking specimen in a medium stage of growth. 🌿 **Figure E:** This Maitake's host is a gnarled oak. 🌿 **Figure F:** These specimens show some color and shape variations.

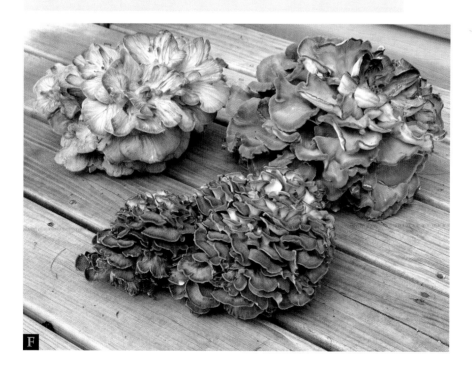

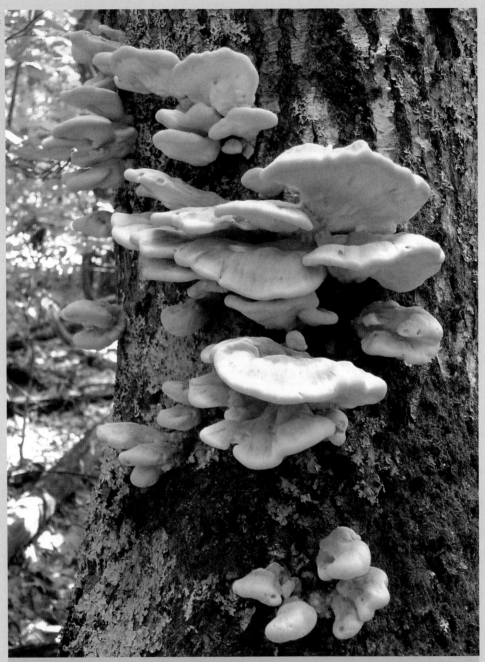

Laetiporus sulphureus at a slightly earlier stage than the specimen shown on opposite page.

Chapter Fifteen

Chicken of the Woods

(Laetiporus sulphureus and *L. cincinnatus)*

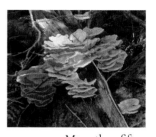

More than fifty pounds of *Laetiporus sulphureus* growing on dead oak, found in early September.

T he Chicken of the Woods is a popular and exceptionally easy-to-recognize mushroom that grows in overlapping clusters or large rosettes. Rosettes can be larger than twenty-four inches across and weigh more than twenty pounds. When found in cluster form on the side of a tree, individual shelves can easily weigh more than one pound each. The size and exceptionally bright colors of this species make it easy to spot from great distance. Many consider it to be a choice edible that tastes somewhat like chicken.

Cap (pileus): The cap measures two to twenty inches across and from one-eighth of an inch to one inch thick. The color of *Laetiporus sulphureus* is from bright orange to salmon or orange-yellow on top with a bright yellow margin. *L. cincinnatus* can have whitish zones on the cap. *L. sulphureus* are usually overlapping, fan-shaped, flat caps that grow as a single shelf or in attached bunches or rosettes on wood. *L. cincinnatus* tends to grow in a rosette at the base of the tree. The color fades toward whitish tones with age. Both species have a pleasant smell.

Tubes (hymenophore): The tubes of *Laetiporus sulphureus* and *L. cincinnatus* are one to four or more millimeters long. The pores of *Laetiporus sulphureus* are minute, angular, and bright sulphur yellow underneath. *L. cincinnatus* has whitish pores.

Stem (stipe): The stem of *Laetiporus sulphureus* is usually short or often broadly attached to the wood. *L. cincinnatus* has a short stem that tends to grow in rosettes at the base of the tree or nearby on the ground.

Flesh: Both species have yellowish white or orangey white flesh.

Spores: The spore print of both species is white.

When and where to find them (ecology): Both species of Chicken of the Woods are most likely found from August through October or later but are sometimes found as early as June. They are very noticeable from a long distance because of their size and very bright colors. They grow on many types of dead or mature trees with hardwoods, such as oak, cherry, or beech, being more likely than conifers. Chicken of the Woods grow very fast. Usually when you find one specimen, there will be many more. Immediately after you remove a younger specimen, it may have a large amount of clear, watery juice that pours—almost like a faucet—out of the specimen and its host. This is a sign that the specimen will be a choice edible.

Preparation: In terms of edibility, Chicken of the Woods can be one of the most variable species. Some collections are tasty and tender, others are not. Do not give up if your first collection is underwhelming. Often with larger specimens, you may only want to use the more tender outer edges of the cap. Be sure to cook thoroughly.

Chicken of the Woods are best sautéed, deep-fried, baked,

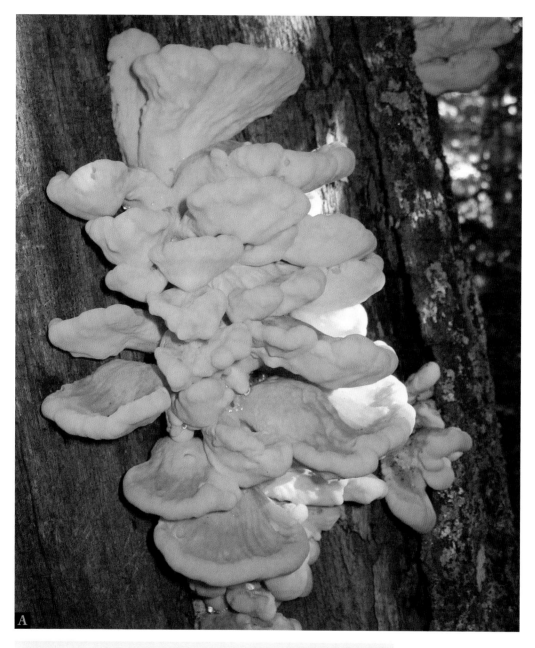

🔖 **Figure A:** This is the same bunch as in Figure G just one day later. Still a bit immature and tender, they have more than doubled in size in twenty-four hours.

and cooked in soups. They can have a lemony, chicken-like taste and texture and go well with chicken or chicken stock. I freeze the specimens after sautéing them. I am still researching drying Chicken of the Woods. Overcooking can make them dry so in most cases, a technique that adds liquid will be better. (If you have ever cooked eggplant and wondered where the oil went, then this will be a similar experience.) Finishing your sauté with cream, chicken, vegetable stock, or a white wine—such as Riesling—is an excellent strategy. Use Chicken of the Woods in alfredo or béchamel-based sauces. Marinating is necessary if you want to grill this species.

The quality of Chicken of the Woods deteriorates if your specimens are too large or mature. Usually smaller thin caps or thick and knobby caps as they first emerge from the wood are better. This species has an unusual texture that becomes sort of woody with age. So how you treat specimens can depend on their age. There is anecdotal evidence that suggests *L. cincinnatus* may be more tender than *L. sulphureus*. A young specimen can be used in many ways and can be refrigerated for a week or more.

Comments: A few people may have sensitivity to Chicken of the Woods so if it is your first time, taste only a small amount. Specimens found growing on conifers should be treated with more caution. Not everyone likes the texture. Some people have mistaken Jack O'Lantern for Chicken of the Woods, which is odd because Chicken of the Woods has pores and Jack O'Lanterns have gills.

Chicken of the Woods can be used for dyeing wool, some fabrics, and paper. When ammonia is used as a mordant, this species will yield an orange color with wool.

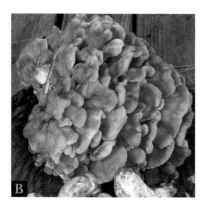

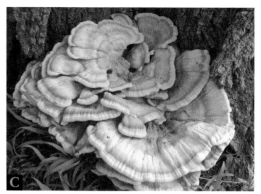

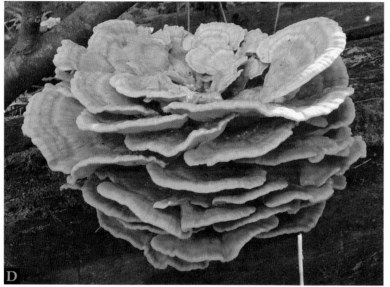

🦃 **Figure B:** The bright color of this *Laetiporus sulphureus* is partly due to being waterlogged, which makes them fairly difficult to cook. Dry sautéing to drive off the water can help. 🦃 **Figure C:** *Laetiporus cincinnatus.* 🦃 **Figure D:** *Laetiporus sulphureus* "rooster." 🦃 **Figure E:** *Laetiporus cincinnatus.*

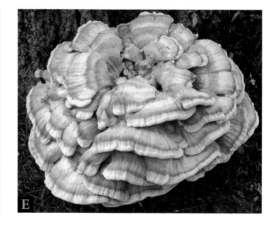

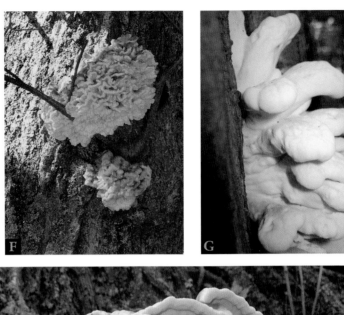

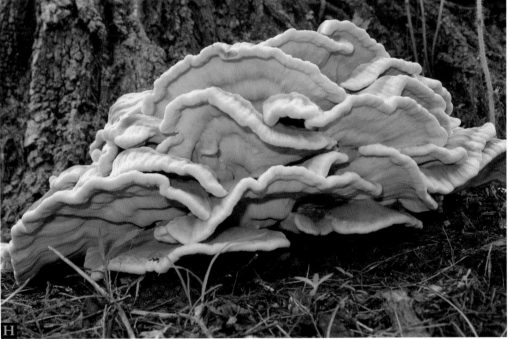

🌿 **Figure F:** *Laetiporus sulphureus.* 🌿 **Figure G:** Newly emerging *Laetiporus sulphureus* will be tender at this point, and they will grow rapidly and still be tender when larger. 🌿 **Figure H:** The whitish underside of *Laetiporus cincinnatus.*

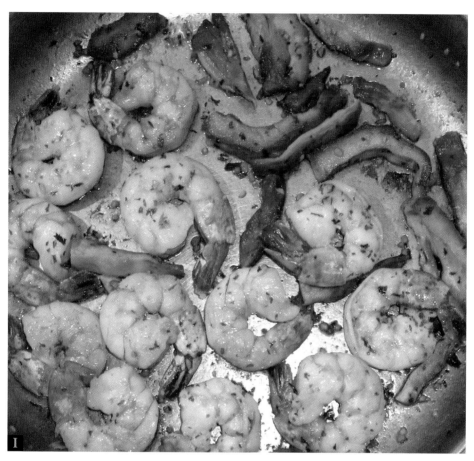

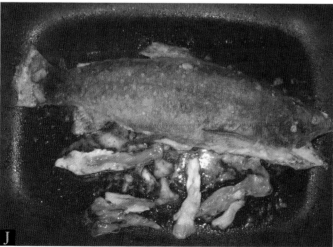

🗡 **Figure I:** Shrimp, *Laetiporus cincinnatus,* parsley, garlic, olive oil, butter, you figure out the rest. Finishing with a Riesling is an excellent option. 🗡 **Figure J:** Large brook trout with *Laetiporus cincinnatus* and Chanterelles.

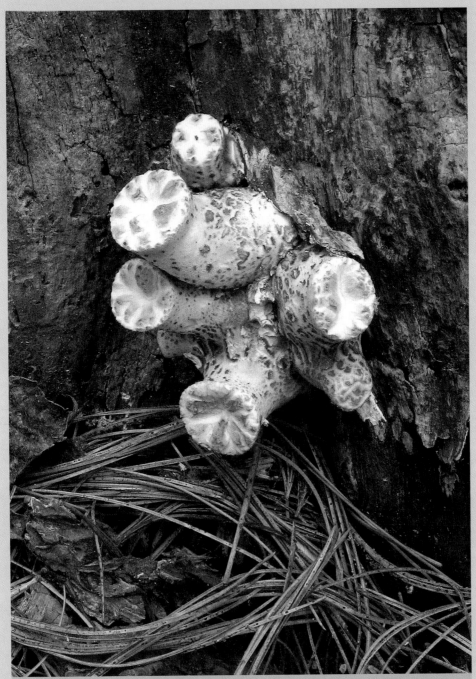

Dryad's Saddle as it first emerges.

Chapter Sixteen

Dryad's Saddle

(Polyporus squamosus)

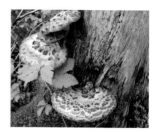

Typical Dryad's
Saddle.

When spring comes around and I cannot find Morels, I am always glad to find some Dryad's Saddle to take home. Also known as Pheasant Back Mushroom, *Polyporus squamosus* has been much maligned as an edible of little value, but I disagree. The difference is in understanding how to pick and cook this species.

Cap (pileus): The cap ranges from two to twelve inches and is circular to kidney- or fan-shaped, thick, and often overlaps on dead wood. It is covered with brown scales that look much like feathers, which is why the species is also called Pheasant Back. The aroma of this species is very distinctive—similar to watermelon rind—and quite pleasant. Although I have seen *Polyporus squamosus* described as mealy, they are not so around here.

Tubes (hymenophore): The tubes may be from one to twelve millimeters long and descend the stalk. The pores are whitish to yellowish tan, small at first, becoming fairly large and angular.

Stem (stipe): The stem is very short, measuring from three-fourths to two inches, and is attached to the wood.

Flesh: Dryad's Saddle has white and nonbruising flesh.

Spores: The spore print is white and is one of the prettiest spore prints that I have printed.

When and where to find them (ecology): This species grows on a variety of very dead hardwoods—especially elm—mostly in May or June but occasionally later. A tree lying on the ground is your best bet. Occasionally specimens may be found on a living tree but the species seems to prefer very dead wood. Wet areas seem to produce more. Dryad's Saddle is quite common and one of only a few decent edibles you will find this time of year. It is a welcome sight to find when Morel hunting is frustrating. *Polyporus squamosus* will be found in the same places each year until the wood is consumed. Although others have called the species just edible or even poor, I find them to be quite tasty. However, specimens must be young; their pore layer needs to be very thin (one-sixteenth of an inch or less); and most importantly, the knife needs to pass through the specimens very easily. I have found that whatever the knife cuts easily is likely to be tender enough for the table. Sometimes the outer edges of a more mature specimen may be tender enough to eat.

Preparation: Once you have found tender specimens, they are best cooked immediately. Like many other wild mushrooms, the aroma of *Polyporus squamosus* often dissipates within hours. Tempura-frying will retain some of the watermelon-like character as will sautéing. Slice specimens thin and cook them hard and fast. Overcooking will create toughness. I have dried this species. They come out as very white, crunchy chips that are tasty to eat in dry form. They retained more of that unique smell than I expected. I have also made a powder with them that looks and smells appetizing. Although the microwave produced something you could make shoes with, I have had luck

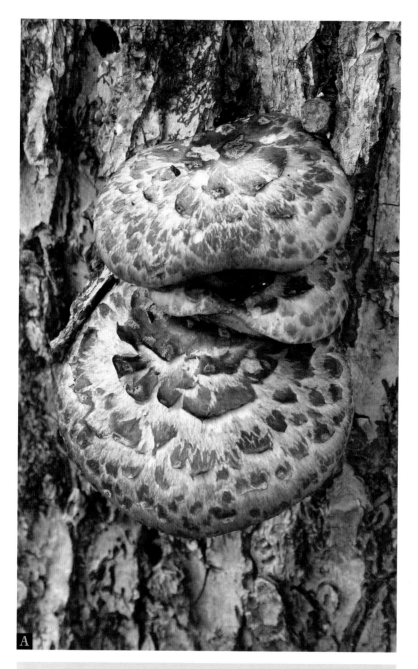

🐾 **Figure A:** Specimens beyond this early stage may be too tough to eat.

with cooking tougher specimens, blending them with chicken stock into the consistency of a smoothie, and then using the mixture to make mushroom soup. Nothing else tastes or smells like this species. I find it quite pleasant when prepared correctly. I could easily identify it by the smell with my eyes closed. Maybe it would taste "mealy" if it was stored in the refrigerator for a couple of days. Actually, because different people perceive smell and taste differently your experience could be different.

Comments: In the spring, Dryad's Saddle is very common. Ignore any specimens that seem leathery and your knife refuses to cut through. Although they resemble Dryad's Saddle, Spring Polypore *(Polyporus arcularius)* and *P. alveolaris* are much smaller and extremely tough.

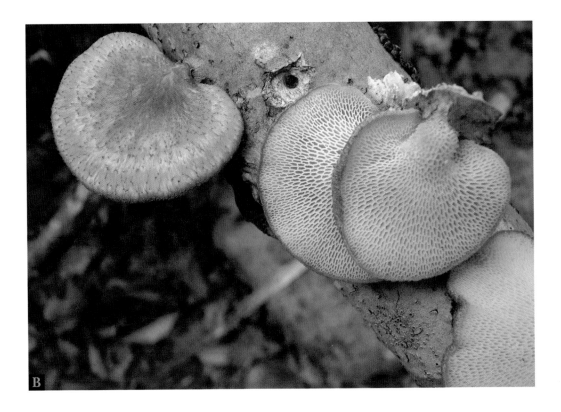

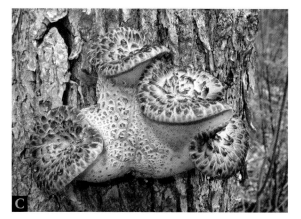

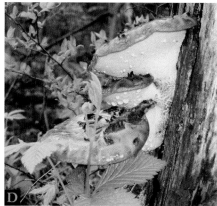

Figure B: *Polyporus alveolaris* has a similar look but is much smaller and very tough. **Figure C:** A young *Polyporus squamosus* with caps beginning to form. **Figure D:** Specimens with droplets on the pore surface. **Figure E:** This is an exceptionally large mature cap. **Figure F:** A close-up of the angular pores. **Figure G:** These are young tender specimens of *Polyporus squamosus*.

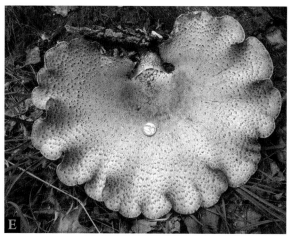

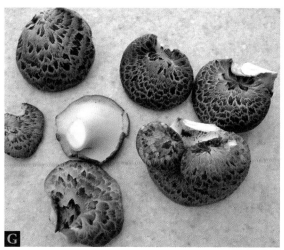

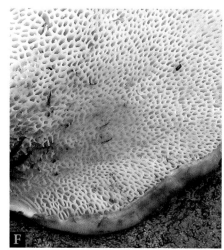

Other Mushrooms

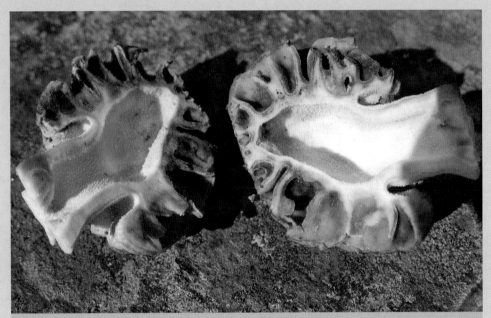
The hollow interior of a Black Morel.

Chapter Seventeen

Yellow Morels and Black Morels

(Morchella esculenta and M. elata)

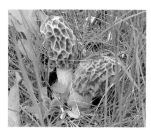

Yellow Morels in the grass and dandelions. Photo by David Guillemette.

Beginning in late April through mid-June, Morels appear in Maine, however, I am not good at finding them. I have not spotted a specimen in several years. Yellow Morels *(Morchella esculenta)* seem to predominate, yet other species are found rarely. No one is sure how many species of Morels exist; but generally they are characterized as Black, Yellow, or Half-free Morels. Black Morels *(Morchella elata)* are likely to appear first, followed by Half-free Morels *(Morchella semilibera),* then Yellow Morels *(Morchella esculenta).* Morels grow throughout the United States.

You must take great care to be absolutely sure that you have not picked the False Morel. They contain a volatile substance known as MMH (monomethyl hydrazine) that is similar to rocket fuel. Some parboil False Morels and do eat them. Do *not* even consider it. There have been numerous poisonings and a few deaths. No False—or even questionable—Morel should *ever* be eaten. I find False Morels throughout my yard as well as in my wood chips and near the red pines.

Fruit body: The fully attached caps of Yellow Morels are yellow, gray, or blond; honeycomb or spongelike; and on a short, sometimes thick, whitish stem. Yellow Morels are normally one to five inches tall; but sometimes, they can be much larger. The fully attached caps of Black Morels have black or brown ridges and tend to be conical, elongated, or bell-shaped. Both species are completely hollow.

Cap (pileus): The Yellow Morel cap is usually conical, oval, bell-shaped, and sometimes quite irregular with grayish or yellowish ribs (never black or dark brown) and darkish to yellow recesses. Normal cap size measures from one to two inches wide and one to four inches tall. The cap looks a bit like a honeycomb or sponge and is never wavy or brain-like. The Black Morel cap is elongated and conical. With dark gray or black ribs and yellow to brown recesses. The bottom of the cap may overhang slightly near the point where it joins to the stem forming a rim. Morels are ascomycetes: They produce spores in sacs, called asci, that are in the recesses on the surface of the cap. No gills or pores are present. The spores of both species are yellow to orange in color.

Stem (stipe): The stem of the Yellow Morel ranges from one to two inches; is whitish, hollow, and usually short with ribs or bumps; and has whitish flesh and a pebbly texture. The stem can become thick with age or have a bulbous base. The stem of the Black Morel measures from one to four inches; is whitish to tan, hollow, and usually short with ribs or bumps; and has whitish flesh and a pebbly texture.

Flesh: The flesh of both species is thin and off white to yellow or brown.

When and where to find them (ecology): Morels grow from as early as late April until about the middle of June. In Maine

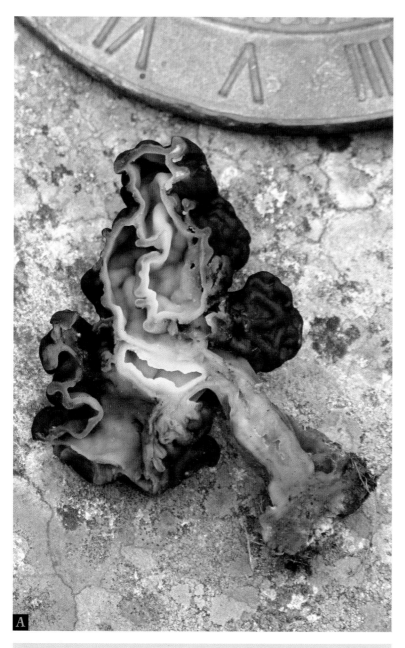

🌿 **Figure A:** False Morel *(Gyromitra esculenta)* is chambered on the inside with an irregular brain-like cap. Very poisonous and sometimes deadly, this species tends to favor pines and other conifers.

Black Morels are likely to appear in May and be found under conifers. Yellow Morels are likely to be found in numbers from late May to late June. Apple orchards are one of the most likely places to find Yellow Morels, usually appearing as the trees start to bloom. Unfortunately, many orchards have been sprayed with pesticides. DDT was applied to the trees from shortly after World War II until it was banned in 1972. Prior to that time trees were sprayed with lead arsenate. The harmful components of these substances persist in the soil for decades. Therefore, Morels found in orchards that have been sprayed may not be safe to eat.

It is safest to find old orchards that are no longer farmed or just old, unmanaged trees. Dead or dying elms are another common host for Morels. Some collectors say to look when the bark is just starting to fall off. Mixed woods with beech, oak, and other hardwoods sometimes support Morels. They may occasionally be found in berry bushes, wood chips, and compost, as well as along field edges, walkways, swimming pools, and gardens. Individual fruit bodies in a patch may exhibit varying shapes and coloration. Some may speak of a gray Morel with light gray ridges and darker recesses, which is actually an immature Yellow Morel.

Preparation: *Never* eat a raw Morel! All Morels contain poisonous volatile constituents and must be cooked thoroughly to be safe to eat. They are delicious sautéed, deep-fried, or dried and reconstituted. One of the best ways to eat Morels is by themselves to appreciate their subtle flavor. Morels cooked with brook trout is a favorite among fishermen. Foods that are not overpowering, such as chicken, fish, cheese, and white sauces, are best with Morels. They make fine soup. Mixing Morels with other mushroom species, especially species of *Agaricus,* may not be the best course.

Comments: In my town I do not know anyone who has found a Morel. I checked every dead elm and old apple tree in town last year with no results. I even checked a burn site even though burn site morels are not known on the east coast. Closer to the coast, where there is a lot of limestone, people find a fair number of Morels. I am guessing the soil has a more neutral ph, whereas, the soil is quite acidic where I live.

Rarely the Half-free Morel *(Morchella semilibera)* is found in April and May. Its cap is attached to the stem halfway up. The Half-free Morel is completely hollow. The Half-free Morel is edible but must be cooked, like all Morels. *Verpa conica* and *V. bohemica,* often known as Thimble Caps, bear a passing resemblance to the Half-free Morel. The cap of these two species of *Verpa* is attached at the very top of the stem like a thimble on the end of a finger. Although some people eat *Verpas,* there have been some poisonings so *Verpas* should be avoided. False Morels *(Gyromitra esculenta)* are usually found in April and May and are quite common. They are poisonous and sometimes deadly and should *never* be eaten. You must be sure to know the differences between Morels and False Morels. False Morel caps are irregular and brain-like with a chambered interior. The caps of true Morels (species of *Morchella*) have a more sponge-like or honeycomb appearance and are completely hollow from top to bottom.

I have attempted to grow some Morel patches around my house, without success so far.

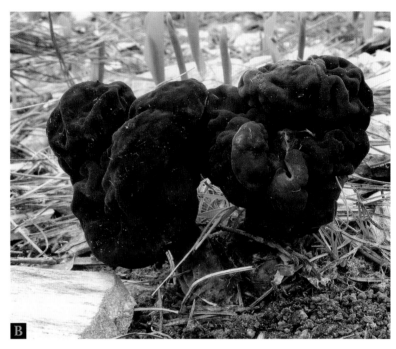

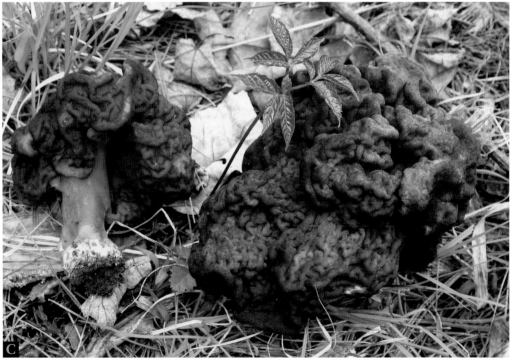

Figure B: False Morels *(Gyromitra esculenta)* like these are poisonous. Figure C: Note the brain-like wavy appearance and color variants of these specimens of False Morel *(Gyromitra esculenta)*, also known as the Conifer False Morel. Figure D: These *Morchella esculenta* were found in a single day. Photo: David Guillemette. Figure E: Species of Morchella are completely hollow from top to bottom usually with a conical or oval attached cap. Note the pebbly texture of the stem both inside and out. Figure F: Morels are occasionally found by garden edges, walkways, swimming pools, and in compost and wood chips. Photo: David Guillemette. Figure G: Shown here is a Yellow Morel with a somewhat grayish appearance. Photo: David Guillemette. Figure H: Yellow Morels from the Central Maine area. Photo: David Guillemette. Figure I: A large collection of Yellow Morels. Photo: David Guillemette.

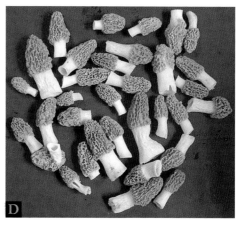

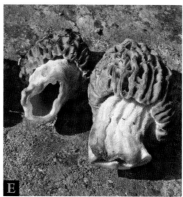

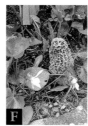

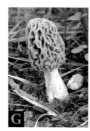

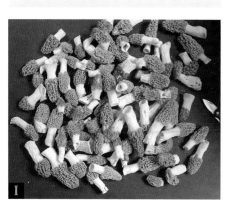

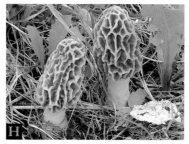

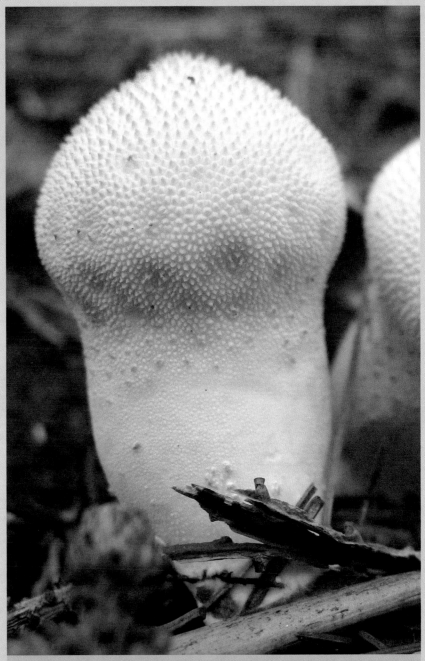

The Gem-studded Puffball *(Lycoperdon perlatum)* is a small, very common edible species.

Chapter Eighteen

Puffballs

(Calvatia gigantea, C. cyathiformis, and Others*)*

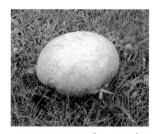

Purple-spored
Puffball *(Calvatia
cyathiformis).*

A Puffball was the first wild mushroom I ever tried. I had heard that if you slice through a Puffball and it is pure white, it would be safe to eat. White all the way through is a very good rule but with a couple of additional precautions you should take. It is best if the Puffball is larger than your fist. Make sure you do not see the pattern of a developing capped mushroom on the inside when you cut open your specimen—you could die from eating an *Amanita* button.

To be safe and if you are a new collector, it is best to stick with the large Puffballs, such as the Giant Puffball *(Calvatia gigantea)* and the Purple-spored Puffball *(C. cyathiformis)*. These two species are big—usually larger than an orange or a grapefruit and often dramatically larger. The largest Puffball ever found was almost four feet across and weighed nearly fifty pounds.

Fruit body: The Giant Puffball *(Calvatia gigantea)* is a large hemispherical fruit, whitish in color, and occasionally found in groups or fairy rings. The Purple-spored Puffball *(C. cyathiformis)* is large, hemispherical, brown in color, and often found in groups. The skin often exhibits shallow cracks.

Stem: *Calvatia gigantea* has no stem, but instead, the species has stringlike attachments to the ground. *C. cyathiformis* has a cup-shaped base firmly attached to the ground. *C. gigantea* will roll easily and there will be very little dirt when you harvest it. *C. cyathiformis* will have dirt attached to the bottom of the stem.

Flesh: Fresh edible examples of either species will have white or whitish flesh all the way through. Giant Puffballs that show yellow to yellowish green interior are past their prime and should not be eaten. Purple-spored Puffballs turn yellowish purple to purple when they are past their prime. Most Puffballs are somewhat soft when you cut into them, like cutting into a loaf of bread. A specimen should not be dense; and if one is very dense, look closely to see if there is an immature mushroom cap developing. If there is, throw the specimen away immediately.

Spores: *Calvatia gigantea* has brownish spores. *C. cyathiformis* has purplish spores as its name suggests.

When and where to find them (ecology): Giant Puffballs can be found usually in late spring or fall among lawns, fields, field edges, and occasionally under hardwoods. Purple-spored Puffballs are found midsummer mostly on lawns or pastures or in very old cemeteries.

Preparation: Puffballs have a pleasant flavor, and I think they are somewhat underrated. Finding one can create a dilemma because a specimen can be quite large and requires fairly immediate preparation. Using a bread knife and slicing them to bread-like thickness or slightly thinner is a good approach. Sautéing or tempura-frying are good techniques. I have a friend who puts slices in his toaster or lightly brushes them with oil and puts them in a toaster oven. I have not tried drying.

Cooking Puffballs in the sauté pan is similar to cooking eggplant in that this species absorbs a lot of oil so if you add too much oil or butter they become soggy. Adding some garlic to the sauté pan is nice. I make small pizzas with them as the "dough," adding tomato sauce or salsa, cheese, and other ingredients. Puffballs can also be substituted for pasta in lasagna or for eggplant or tofu. Freeze precooked slices of Puffballs between sheets of plastic wrap for later use.

Comments: Puffballs are some of the easiest species of mushrooms to identify. A Giant Puffball that is the size of a soccer ball is not uncommon. They appear very quickly and are a surprise to see. You might easily think that a child lost a ball. Most species are edible; however, Pigskin Puffballs that have a black interior should *never* be eaten.

Consider throwing any Puffballs that are past their prime into your yard or woods. This will distribute the spores, and with some luck, a few specimens may grow.

Both *Calvatia gigantean* and *C. cyathiformis* can be used to dye wool, textiles, and paper. Using ammonia as a mordant, *C. gigantea* creates a red-brown color and *C. cyathiformis* yields a rust red color.

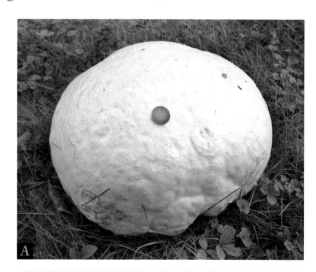

Figure A: Giant Puffball *(Calvatia gigantea).*

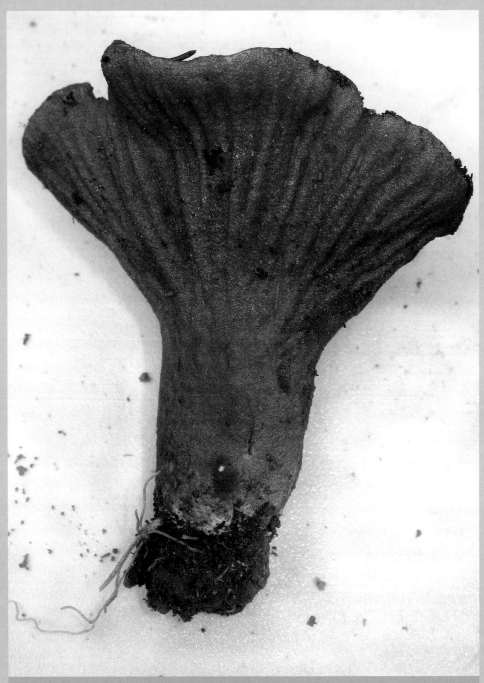

A typical Lobster Mushroom.

Chapter Nineteen

Lobster Mushroom

(Hypomyces lactifluorum)

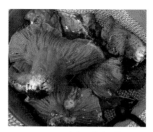

A hatful of Lobster Mushrooms.

From their color that is similar to cooked lobster meat or lobster shell, you can see why this species is called the Lobster Mushroom. In addition, when cooked, this species can have a seafood-like aroma. However, the Lobster Mushroom is actually an example of a mold attacking a mushroom. *Hypomyces lactifluorum* attacks and parasitizes *Lactarius piperatus* or *Russula brevipes* and covers the entire fruit body with an orange skin. *Lactarius piperatus* has a peppery flavor that is improved by *Hypomyces*. *Russula brevipes,* which has very crumbly flesh, becomes dense and less breakable.

Cap (pileus): The cap is that of the *Russula* or *Lactarius* it parasitizes. *Russula* and *Lactarius* genera can develop a concave cap and the Lobster Mushroom may look somewhat like that. *Hypomyces lactifluorum* mold may seriously deform the shape and be very irregular.

Stem (stipe): The stem of the Lobster Mushroom is usually quite short and shaped like the mushroom it parasitizes.

Flesh: The flesh of the *Hypomyces lactifluorum* is white or slightly orangey white and quite dense.

Spores: The spores are colorless and difficult to collect.

When and where to find them (ecology): Lobster Mushrooms can be found under a wide variety of hardwoods and conifers, especially hemlock. You will generally find the most specimens during September and October, but they can appear as early as July or August. Any place where *Russula brevipes* or *Lactarius piperatus* grows, you may find the Lobster Mushroom. They are often very noticeable but will occasionally be partially underground just barely breaking the soil. No other mushroom looks remotely like them.

Preparation: There are often deep cracks in the surface of the caps of Lobster Mushrooms. The caps may collect dirt as they come out of the ground and cleaning them can be difficult. If dirt has collected in the cracks, the specimens can rapidly spoil. *Hypomyces lactifluorum* can be highly variable in their flavor characteristics. Fresh specimens that are completely white on the interior are best. However, they can tend to have brown spots that should be trimmed off. Lobster mushrooms match well with white wine. Clean, young specimens will often have a seafood odor as you sauté them and would be a natural accompaniment to lobster, crab, or other seafood. If overcooked the seafood-like flavor may dissipate. Plain preparation, such as sautéing and tempura-frying, is a good choice, and the rendered orange-colored juice adds to the presentation of the dish. They can be successfully dried. This species is often delicious, but older, darker orange specimens may be somewhat mealy.

Comments: Some mushroom field guides have suggested that *Hypomyces lactifluorum* could attack a poisonous mushroom, such as an *Amanita,* and cause poisoning. However, there does not seem to be much actual evidence of this. People have eaten Lobster Mushrooms for hundreds of years with few known incidents. As always, though, if you have never eaten a particular type of mushroom, try a small amount first. In my experience, this species is highly variable in flavor. An older specimen often starts to smell because of rot spots that develop from dirt sitting on the top or in crevices of the cap. They are quite often infested with maggots. Do not give up if you find a specimen that is not edible. You can still break or slice it up and distribute the pieces where species of *Russula* and *Lactarius* grow and perhaps you will find more Lobster Mushrooms there the next year.

Lobster Mushrooms can be used for dyeing wool, some fabrics, and paper. When ammonia is used as a mordant, they will yield a cinnamon pink to red color.

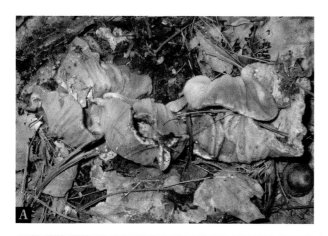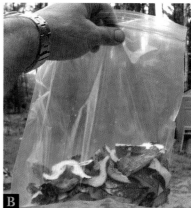

❧ **Figure A:** *Hypomyces lactifluorum* get dirty and moldy with rot spots if they are a bit old. ❧ **Figure B:** I spread Lobster Mushroom slices like these where species of *Lactarius* and *Russula* grow on my property.

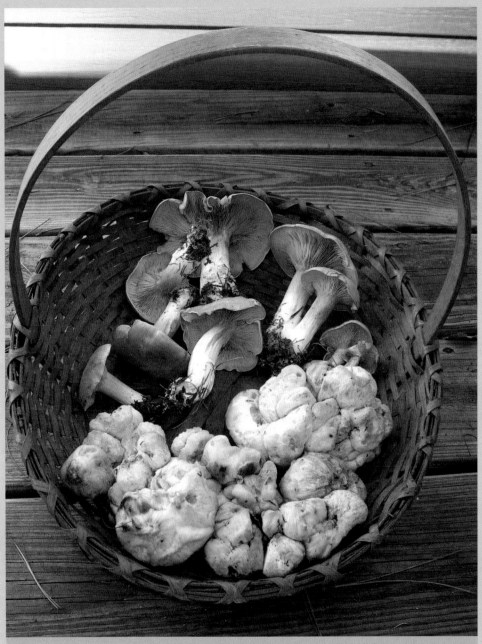

A collection of aborted and non-aborted forms with pink spores
evident on one of the caps.

Chapter Twenty

Aborted Entoloma

(Entoloma abortivum)

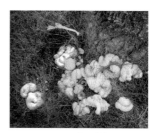

A healthy group
of aborted fruit
bodies.

The middle of September brings on the Aborted Entoloma and its intimately related companion the Honey
Mushroom. The interaction of the mycelia of these
species creates an aborted fruit body that somewhat resembles
a Puffball. However, the fruit body of the Aborted Entoloma is
more bumpy and irregular in shape. The Aborted Entoloma is
one of my favorites to find, and I have enjoyed the species for
more than twenty years. When found at the right time and prepared correctly, specimens are excellent.

Although the rules for collecting say to avoid *Entolomas,* the
Aborted Entoloma is a special case because it resembles no other
species of *Entoloma*. The Aborted Entoloma has no gills so it is
easy to identify.

There is some controversy surrounding this species and its
relationship with the Honey Mushroom (*Armillaria mellea*) complex. Originally, mycologists believed that Honey Mushrooms
parasitize and deform the *Entoloma* fruit body. Today, many
mycologists say the *Entoloma* parasitizes the Honey Mushroom
and that the deformed mushroom is actually an aborted Honey
Mushroom. I often wonder if this is something that could go
either way, depending on which mycelium is "stronger." I have
found fruit bodies with two very different looks to them. Keep

in mind that this is my personal speculation and that I have no scientific proof. However, it is certainly possible that different types of Honey Mushrooms would abort differently. The Honey Mushrooms on conifer stumps that are near my house are *Armillaria ostoyae*. The fruit bodies of both the Honey Mushroom and the Aborted Entoloma were large and abundant in 2007. Tom Volk, a renowned mushroom scientist, thinks the aborted fruit bodies should be called *Aborted Armillaria*. He is likely to be right. Both the aborted and non-aborted forms of the *Entoloma* are usually found together along with Honey Mushrooms. Occasionally Honey Mushrooms in their non-aborted form are not present.

Cap (pileus): The cap of the non-aborted form measures from one to five inches diameter; is gray or gray-tan in color; and is convex and round to somewhat kidney-shaped, with inrolled edges that become flat or upturned with age. There can be a slight hint of pink on the cap.

The cap of the aborted form ranges from one-half of an inch to four inches and is whitish, bumpy, and usually depressed or folded at the center. Gills are not present. The cap shape can be highly variable: Often it will have splits at or near the center. Although it can look somewhat like a Puffball, the cap of the aborted form is usually too deformed to be too similar. The cap of the aborted form can also look folded or twisted and almost brain-like. The white color on the outside rubs off easily, revealing some tannish tones.

Gills (hymenophore): The gills of the non-aborted form are grayish at first—developing pink tones with age—and attached, running down the stalk a bit (see Figure E). Gills are not present in the aborted fruits.

Stem (stipe): The stem of the non-aborted form ranges from one to four inches long and from one-fourth to one-half of an inch thick, with the length usually corresponding roughly to the width of the cap. The stem is often slightly enlarged at the base. The stem of the aborted form is often short and usually somewhat brownish and striated, or it is almost stemless.

Flesh: The flesh is whitish in the gilled form of *Entoloma* and fairly dense and meaty. The flesh of the aborted form is somewhat pithy inside and can have pinkish tones and may bruise slightly pink. Sometimes there are air spaces in the interior of

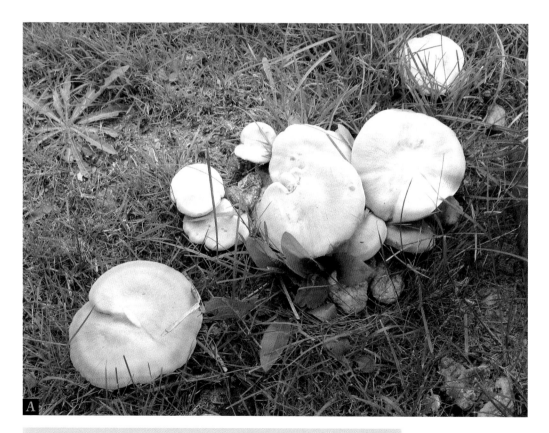

🔖 **Figure A:** These are gilled, non-aborted fruit bodies.

the aborted form. There can be brown rot spots inside older specimens where cracks in the cap have allowed water, dirt, or bugs to enter. The aborted fruit bodies do absorb water readily so they require careful cleaning to avoid becoming waterlogged.

Spores: The non-aborted gilled fruit has pink spores.

When and where to find them (ecology): *Entolomas* are found mostly from mid-September through October and coincide with the onset of heavy *Armillaria* growth and are quite common. *Entoloma abortivum* is saprobic and usually found around rotting wood, wood chips, stumps, and under older diseased trees around the roots. Often found in lawns and parks and some woodland locations, *Entolomas* seem to favor very rotten wood. They will be found in the same location year after year until the wood is consumed. The aborted fruit bodies are most often in big bunches with the gilled form growing right with them or nearby. Honey Mushrooms are also likely to be present.

Preparation: I have eaten the gilled version and they are quite good, but beginners should avoid them because they resemble other *Entolomas* that may be poisonous. Pick only the aborted fruits. There are usually more than enough when you find them so bypassing the gilled specimens is easy.

The aborted fruit has a spotty reputation as an edible that I feel is undeserved. However, they must be collected and cooked correctly. Look for fruits that are quite white, have few or no cracks in the top, and feel relatively dense (not spongy). Being a bit pithy on the inside is actually normal. It is best to avoid specimens with brown spots, and waterlogged specimens are hard to cook. They are occasionally wormy so also check closely for small white maggots. Be very careful until you are sure of your ability to identify safely as you do not want to mistake the aborted fruit for button-stage *Amanitas* that can be deadly. *Amanitas* will have lines indicating a developing fruit and are much denser inside and smooth on the outside. Do *not* take a chance.

Sometimes a small part of the fruit will be spoiling a bit while another part is quite nice and requires trimming. Cut the stem off. Clean them very carefully as they can hold bits of grit quite frequently. The pithy nature of the interior can cause them to absorb water. Do not let them get waterlogged. These are very good sautéed and my rule is "cook them hard." I believe that their spotty reputation as an edible is due to undercooking. I like to cut them in half from side to side. They are best when they are well-browned and have most of the moisture cooked out and reclaimed, which will reduce their size by more than half. They have a really pleasant nutty flavor. They are only fair deep-fried. You also may have bad luck with these in a stir-fry or with other mixing strategies unless they are the first item you cook or they are partially precooked before adding to the mix. The flavor is somewhat subtle so mixing with strong-flavored foods may cause the flavor to be lost. I like them best sautéed.

Comments: As with any species tried for the first time it is best to try a small bit first. When you cannot absolutely identify a specimen, be safe and throw it out. Beginning collectors should avoid eating the gilled version. *Entolomas* can be very difficult to identify and other species of *Entoloma* can be poisonous. The Honey Mushrooms that grow around them are edible for most people but these are probably best avoided, too, because some people have reactions to them. *Armillaria* is a complex rather than a single species, making absolute identification fairly difficult. Anecdotal evidence suggests that *Armillaria* growing around conifer stumps are more likely to offend. In any case, this species is not for beginners. Generally, I do not eat Honey Mushrooms. With so much around to eat at this time of year, bypassing them is easy.

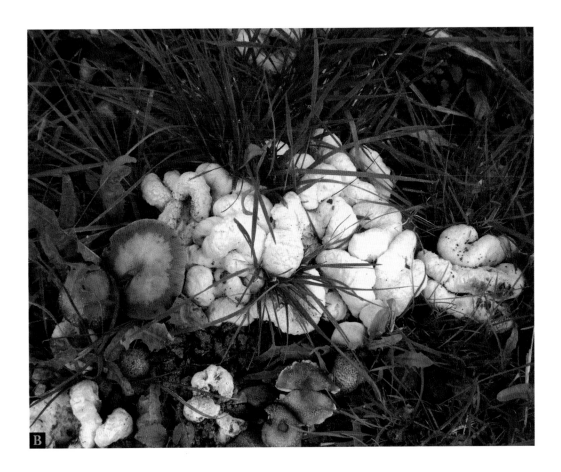

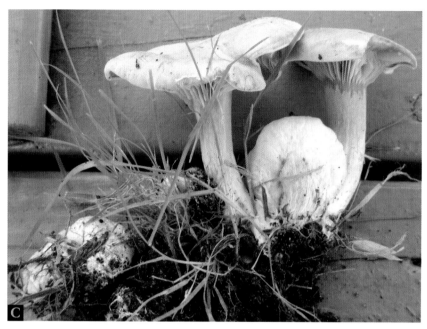

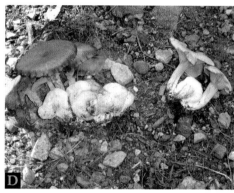

Figure B: *Armillaria* fruit bodies are growing next to the aborted form of the *Entolomas*. **Figure C:** The gilled form of Entoloma (non-aborted) intimately joined to an Aborted Entoloma. **Figure D:** More *Armillaria-Entoloma* relationships. **Figure E:** Gill attachment of the non-aborted form. **Figure F:** Honey Mushrooms joined at the base with aborted fruit bodies.

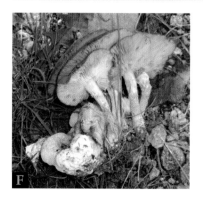

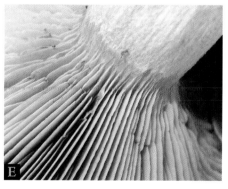

Section Five

Medicinal Mushrooms

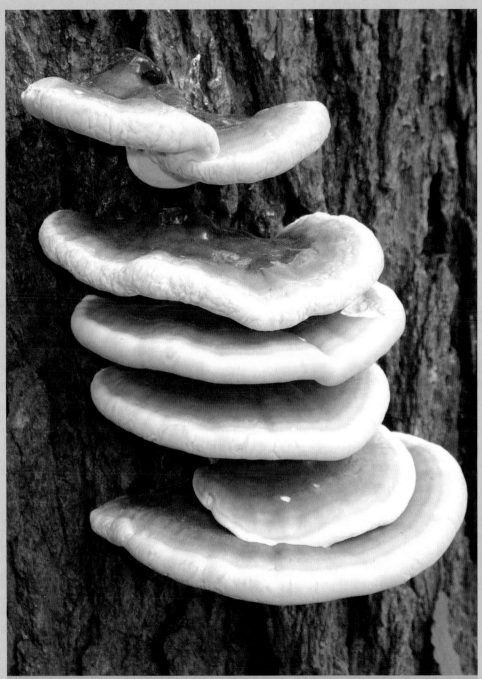

Ganoderma tsugae at about fifty percent of full size.

Chapter Twenty-one

Reishi

(Ganoderma tsugae and *G. lucidum)*

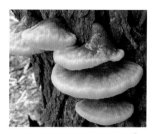

Nice group of *Ganoderma tsugae* on eastern hemlock.

G*anoderma tsugae,* the Hemlock Reishi Mushroom, is quite common in central Maine and elsewhere in the Northeast. It grows on dead or dying eastern hemlock, a very common tree. This species is very showy, exhibiting bright red colors and a varnished look that darkens with maturity. *G. tsugae* contains protein-bound polysaccharides, which are known to have medicinal properties. Looking nearly identical to *G. tsugae, G. lucidum* grows on hardwoods but is very rare in this region.

Cap (pileus): The cap of both species measures from one and one-half to fifteen inches across and from one-half of an inch to one and one-half inches thick. The cap is knobby at first; has whitish tan to orange tones, becoming deep red; and fan- or kidney-shaped with zones. The cap can have a varnished appearance. The margin (edge) may be yellow-tan or whitish. At maturity, the cap becomes covered with the brown spores.

Tubes (hymenophore): The tubes range from one-eighth to three-eighths of an inch thick, and the interior of the pore layer is brown in *Ganoderma tsugae* and may be lighter in *G. lucidum.* At the surface the pores of *G. tsugae* and *G. lucidum* are whitish to light tan with four to six pores per millimeter.

Stem (stipe): The stem of both species ranges from nonexistent and broadly attached to the side of a tree, to several inches long and angled if growing from a stump or root.

Flesh: In *Ganoderma tsugae* the flesh is whitish and often bruises brownish when cut. In *G. lucidum* the flesh is brown.

Spores: Both species have brown spores.

When and where to find them (ecology): *Ganoderma tsugae* is found on dead or dying eastern hemlock but may grow on other conifers beginning in late May or early June and continue into July or in the fall. Trees that woodpeckers have been working on in shadier locations are a likely location. Woodpeckers are probable suspects in the transmission of spores/mycelium from tree to tree. Specimens will be found on the side of a tree or occasionally growing on the ground from a root or on top of a stump. They will grow on the same tree for many years. *G. lucidum* grows in similar fashion on hardwoods.

Preparation: Mushroom field guide author Bill Russell brought it to my attention that the tender edges of *Ganoderma tsugae* are edible when they first emerge. *G. tsugae* is not well known as an edible and most field guides list it as inedible. They may be harvested when they are a whitish to tan knob with no orange, red, or varnish showing yet. The fruit body grows back in the same season if you do not cut it too close. *G. tsugae* is really quite tasty when sautéed with oil and butter.

Powder or thin slices of the dried fruit body can be made into a tincture or liquor. A tincture can be made using alcohol, such as eighty- or one-hundred-proof vodka, and water. To make the tincture: Fill up a container, such as a bottle or jar, at least halfway with dried powder then add vodka until it reaches the top of the container. Let the mixture sit for a few days or up to two weeks. Strain off the liquid and pour it through an unbleached coffee filter. Squeeze the mash (marc) to get as much of the liquid as possible, which yields a single extraction. You may take the leftover single-extracted mash and boil it (decoct) for two hours or more in water. Reduce the liquid by half and add it to your first extraction making a stronger double extraction maintaining an alcohol concentration of around twenty-five percent. Chris Hobbs's *Medicinal Mushrooms: An Exploration of Tradition, Healing, & Culture* covers this process in

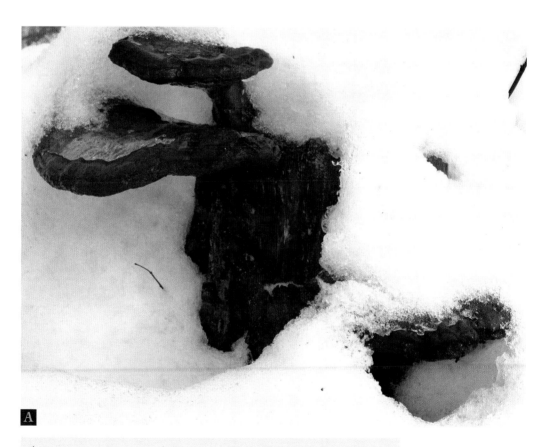

A

🔥 **Figure A:** A few specimens were found during the off-season.

detail. The powder can also be steeped into a tea, which is pleasant but quite bitter. So it requires a bit of sweetening to be palatable. The tincture/liquor is quite assertive with a slightly medicinal flavor and reminds me of scotch whiskey. A bit of sweetness may help here, too. Both tinctures and teas will have a pleasant reddish color.

Recently, I made some English-style ale, using ground fruit bodies as a replacement for bittering hops. My first batch was a bit too bitter. My second batch was quite successful when used with amber ale malt. It added a very slight hint of reddish color to the finished product. Two to three heaping tablespoons per five-pound can of malt is about right for a medium to heavy ale like India pale ale or strong ale.

The dried fruit bodies of both species can also be ground up for use. Running them through a hand-crank meat grinder is hard work, though, similar to grinding a piece of rubber or foam insulation. Place any pieces that pass through the grinder in rubbery little chunks into the blender and chop them further. However, big pieces of the dried specimens may kill your blender. Some opt to slice them thinly for preparation.

Comments: As always try a small bit first. The medicinal properties of the two species have a long history in Chinese medicine. *Ganoderma tsugae* is known as *Songshan Lingzhi* by the Chinese. More recent scientific studies indicate that both *G. tsugae* and *G. lucidum* may be useful in treating some types of cancers, especially breast cancer. *G. tsugae* has been found to have similar properties to *G. lucidum*. Much of the medicinal value may be concentrated in the extremely tough rubbery stem. If you have health issues or take medication there is a possibility of interaction. Check with your doctor.

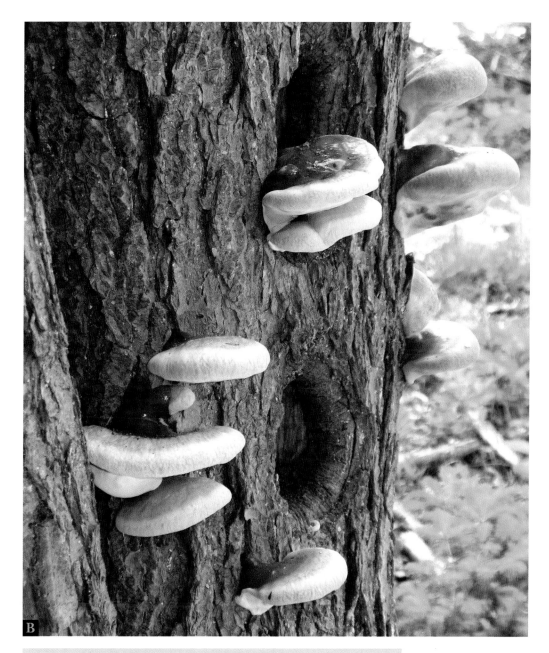

🐾 **Figure B:** *Ganoderma tsugae* at about twenty-five percent of full size.

Ganoderma tsugae can be used for dyeing wool, some fabrics, and paper. Anne William's experimentation reveals that this species will yield a rust color when ammonia is used as a mordant with wool.

When you find either species, you may have to wait for several weeks for the fruits to reach full size. Because you will likely be monitoring the specimens for a while, some patch maintenance is a good idea. Kill any slugs you see in the area and try to brush off any other bugs that may be eating your specimens. Because they are often on trees with woodpecker holes, sawdust often falls on top of the cap that should be brushed or blown off. Small plants growing nearby may need to be weeded or trimmed so that the fruit body does not end up with grasses, stems, or twigs growing through the cap as you can see in the following bunchberry photograph (see Figure D). It is best not to remove any shading plants.

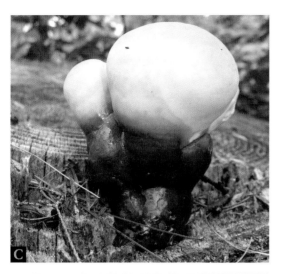

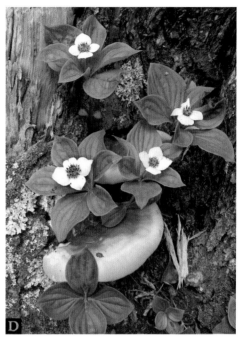

Figure C: Button stage and early growth. **Figure D:** *Ganoderma tsugae* and bunchberry. **Figure E:** *Ganoderma tsugae* showing the white pores. **Figure F:** At this early stage, emerging knobs may be cut for consumption.

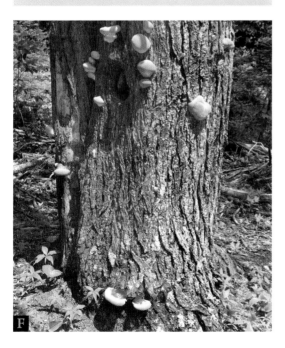

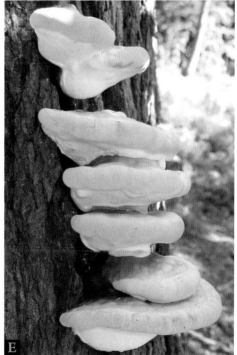

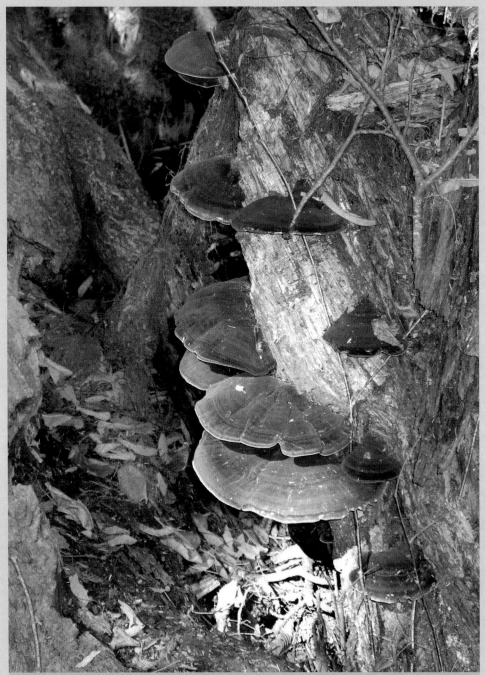

Young and fresh specimen of Artist's Conk.

Chapter Twenty-two

Artist's Conk

(Ganoderma applanatum)

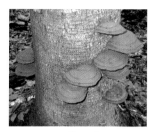

Ganoderma applanatum on birch.

Artist's conk is exceptionally common in Maine, growing on older sugar maples and many other hardwood trees. This species often persists for many years. When picked, the interior flesh of Artist's Conk reveals layers of tubes that are like rings on on the inside of a tree trunk. There is scientific evidence developing that indicates this mushroom has antibacterial properties.

Artists use fresh *Ganoderma applanatum* to etch designs on and dried specimens as "canvases" to paint landscapes and other types of paintings. These renderings can be displayed differently than most paintings because the mushroom will stand on its side on a table or shelf. Eventually, the specimens become almost as hard as a block of wood and will last for many years.

Cap (pileus): The cap ranges from four to twenty-four inches across and from fan- or kidney-shaped to slightly convex to hoof-shaped. The cap can have zones, bumps, lines, and cracks and is exceptionally hard especially after the first year. The cap is usually gray in the off-season and brown in the summer when covered with spores. As it ages, it can become several inches thick.

Tubes (hymenophore): A new layer of tubes that measures from one-eighth to one-half of an inch thick is built each suc-

173

cessive year. The tubes are brown. The pores are white, four to six per millimeter, and bruise to brown when touched or bruised except in winter.

Stem (stipe): The stem is not present and the specimen is broadly attached to the wood.

Flesh: The flesh is very hard and brown or brown and white.

Spores: The spores are brown and tend to collect on the top of the cap in summer.

When and where to find them (ecology): One of the most common shelf mushrooms to see, the Artist's Conk is very easy to find on mature or dead hardwood. Near streams can often be an ideal place to look because that tends to have more dead wood and be a moist microclimate. Sugar maples that are on their way out are very likely to be infected with *Ganoderma applanatum*. This species has a strong but pleasant woodsy smell.

Preparation: Artist's conk is too tough and woody to be edible but can be made into a tea or tincture. As always, try a small amount at first. If you have health issues or take medication, there is a possibility of interaction so be sure to check with your doctor. Artist's conk contains polysaccharides and triterpenoids that have various medicinal implications. *Ganoderma applanatum* can be made into a medicinal tea by drying thoroughly and grinding with a meat grinder or other type of grinder. But I do not recommend you use a blender.

Comments: If collecting for artwork, please note that specimens need to be removed very carefully. They can be exceptionally difficult to remove and you may need a hatchet for a harder older specimen, but you can often push down hard from the top to loosen an Artist's Conk. You may have to push in several places, and it is best if the specimen does not come off all at once and fall to the ground because it can bruise or scratch easily. Instead, try to ease it off. You should not touch the pore surface in any way or it will bruise and damage the surface. Be careful so that you also carry and store a specimen so that the pores touch nothing.

While still fresh, you can use techniques similar to conventional dry point etching for a sepia-colored design on your specimen; or after drying, when the pore surface becomes hard and is not so delicate, your specimen may be painted. However, if you pick Artist's Conk in winter, the pore surface will be hard and will not be successfully etched, but it can still be painted.

Artist's Conk has a strong, fragrant smell. For some reason, cats can be too interested in the smell of fresh specimens.

Artist's Conk can be used for dyeing wool, some fabrics, and paper. When ammonia is used as a mordant, this species will yield a rust color with wool.

The Red-belted Polypore (*Fomitopsis pinicola*) is also quite common and looks like Artist's Conk. However, *Fomitopsis pinicola* often has darker blackish or green tones on the cap and a red or maroon band near the outer margin. The Red-belted Polypore has whitish flesh and white spores. Usually found on pine or hemlock, this species sometimes grows on hardwoods. *Fomitopsis pinicola* can be quite large and thick and may be used as a "canvas," too. But this species bruises, etches are more yellowish, and its pores often yellow somewhat when dried.

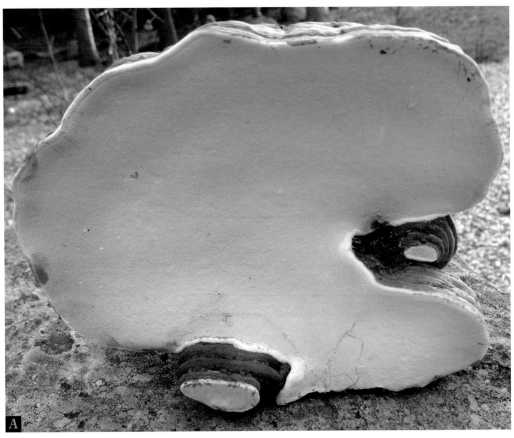

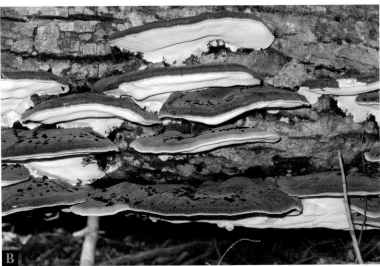

❧ **Figure A:** *Ganoderma applanatum* showing the white pores. ❧ **Figure B:** Young fresh *Ganoderma applanatum* are very brown because of heavy sporulation in summer. ❧**Figure C:** These specimens are perfect for artwork. ❧ **Figure D:** A fresh Artist's Conk turns brown wherever scratched or scored. Once the specimen dries out, it becomes very hard and the artwork becomes permanent. Art by Jody King. ❧**Figure E:** This Red-belted Polypore measures about fifteen inches across and is growing on a very dead pine. Note the red "belt" at the edge of the cap.

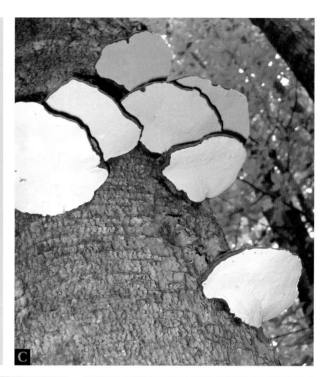

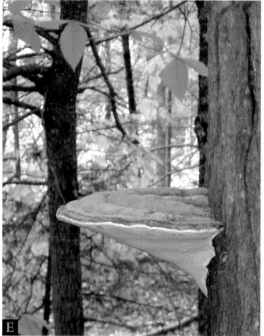

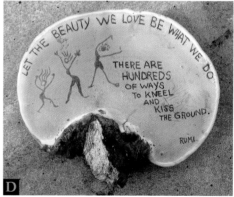

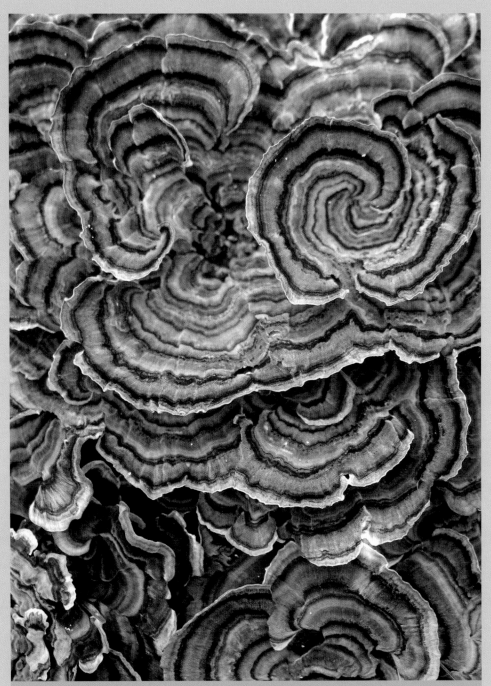

The Turkey Tail's interesting color variations.

Chapter Twenty-three

Turkey Tail

(Trametes versicolor)

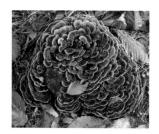

A stump is completely engulfed by *T. versicolor.*

The Turkey Tail is possibly the most common mushroom you will find. Saprobic, this species grows everywhere on dead or rotting stumps and branches. As *versicolor* suggests, specimens are quite variable in color. Because they are so beautiful, Turkey Tails are often used for decorative purposes. Specimens dry easily and become leathery tough. I have seen the Turkey Tail used by artists in various assemblages and even as jewelry. The species can also be used to make blue and green dyes for wool and other fabrics. There has been substantive research conducted regarding the medicinal value of the Turkey Tail as adjunct cancer treatment for colorectal cancer and leukemia. In fact, a protein-bound polysaccharide, called PSK (Krestin), has been developed in Japan for adjunct cancer therapy.

Cap (pileus): The cap measures from one-half of an inch to four inches across and is flat or wavy, overlapping, leathery, and thin. The cap is finely hairy, with zones of different colors—such as blue, green, rust, and brown—with a whitish margin often in rosettes, and is semicircular, fan-, or kidney-shaped.

Tubes (hymenophore): The tubes are very shallow ranging from less than one to three millimeters. The pores are exceptionally small (three or more pores per millimeter) and they are white or yellowish with age.

Stem (stipe): This species has no stem and is broadly attached to the wood.

Flesh: The flesh of the Turkey Tail is thin, leathery, and white.

Spores: The spores are white.

When and where to find them (ecology): Turkey Tails are located everywhere on dead wood and stumps from September to December but occasionally earlier. They may persist on a stump or log for two or three years.

Preparation: As always, try a small amount at first. If you have health issues or take medication, there is a possibility of interaction so be sure to check with your doctor. Pick young clean specimens with very white pore surfaces. To clean specimens, you may want to cut off the edges that were attached to the wood with scissors. This species can be dried, ground, and decocted to make a tea or tincture. The tea is fairly pleasant.

A tincture can be made using alcohol, such as eighty- or one-hundred-proof vodka, and water. To make the tincture: Fill a container, such as a bottle or jar, at least halfway with dried Turkey Tail powder, then add vodka until it reaches the top of the container. Let the mixture sit for a few days or up to two weeks. Strain off the liquid and pour it through an unbleached coffee filter. Squeeze the filter after it has stopped dripping. This process yields a single extraction. You may take the left-over single-extracted mash (marc) and boil it (decoct) in water. Reduce the liquid by half and add it to your first extraction making a stronger double extraction maintaining an alcohol concentration of around twenty-five percent. Chris Hobbs's *Medicinal Mushrooms: An Exploration of Tradition, Healing, & Culture* covers this process in detail.

Comments: This mushroom is also known as *Coriolus versicolor.* In this area of the Northeast, predominantly blue fruit bodies are common. The Turkey Tail can resemble *Trichaptum biformis,* the Velvet-toothed Polypore, which has violet tones and a violet-tinged, toothy underside. Watch for other look-alikes: False Turkey Tail *(Stereum ostria)* is more petal-shaped, hairy, with russet or brownish zones, and a brownish underside. *Trametes hirsuta* is whitish or gray and hairy. Parchment fungi are much smaller than the Turkey Tails. Turkey Tails rot wood very quickly and aggressively and can become a problem for mushroom farmers by infecting logs inoculated with another species.

Turkey Tails can be used for dyeing wool, some fabrics, and paper. When ammonia is used as a mordant, the species will yield a brown color with wool.

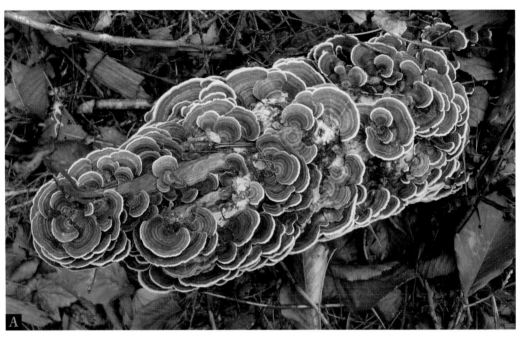

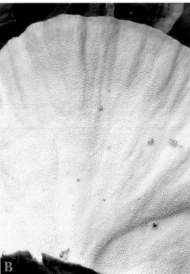

🐾 **Figure A:** *T. versicolor* with blue tones. 🐾 **Figure B:** Underneath, the cap is very white with barely discernable pores. 🐾 **Figure C:** Turkey Tails do not mind sharing this substrate with *Pyncnoporus cinnabarinus*, the Cinnabar-red Polypore. 🐾 **Figure D:** A closer view of Turkey tails and the Cinnabar-red Polypore, *Pyncnoporus cinnabarinus*.

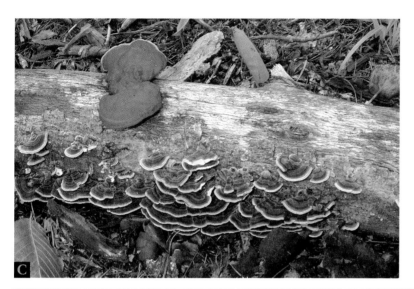

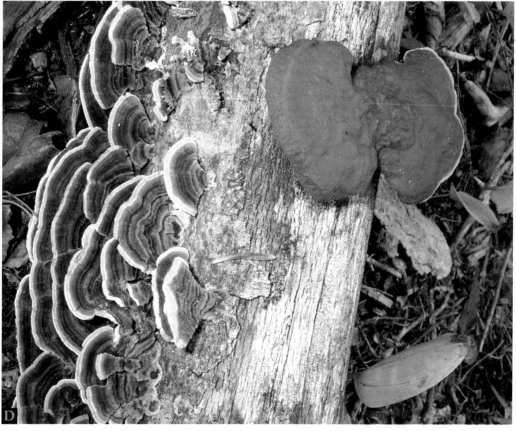

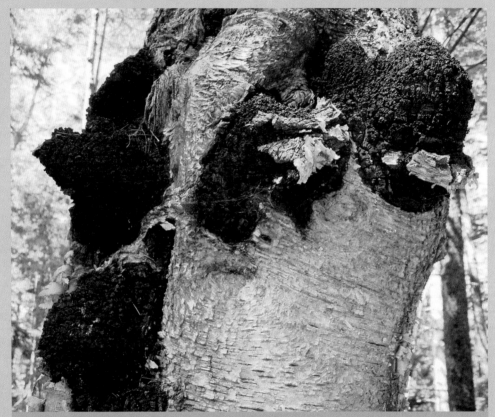

Chaga cankers on a mostly dead yellow birch.

Chapter Twenty-four

Chaga

(Inonotus obliquus)

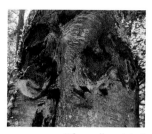

The yellow birch after removing the Chaga.

Many people do not immediately recognize Chaga, also known as Clinker Polypore, as a fungus. For example, a person recently told me that she had seen Chaga before but thought the specimens were a bug infestation. Rather than being mushroomlike, Chaga is a large black canker. It is dense, very hard, and deeply cracked on the surface, resembling something that has been burned. Sometimes, hints of the yellow interior can be seen. Chaga often gets its start on a scarred birch.

Flesh: The interior is yellow to yellow-brown, often with some bits of white mixed in, and is moderately hard with a somewhat pebbly, corky texture. The outer surface is dark brown to black, very hard, and has a deeply cracked texture that is quite brittle with pieces easily rubbing or falling off.

When and where to find them (ecology): Chaga can be found all year because it persists on the tree for many years. It is most often found on yellow or white birch. It is probably possible to find it on gray birch but gray birch is more likely to be infected with *Piptoporus betulina,* the Birch Polypore. Because gray and white birch occasionally hybridize in this region, exact identification of the tree can be difficult. Chaga has been reported to grow also on hardwoods, such as beech or hornbeam; but I have never found a specimen on any tree except birch. Current information suggests that Chaga found on birch has the best medicinal qualities.

Chaga can be easier to find in the winter because birches are easier to spot and because the Chaga often grows high on the tree where the greenery may obscure the specimens during the warmer months. A hatchet or axe is usually required to remove Chaga, which can be easier to remove when frozen. Scarred trees created by excavating or skidding logs during lumber harvesting can develop Chaga. Older trees are more likely to be infected although specimens can be found on middle-aged trees as well.

Preparation: As always, try a small amount at first. If you have health issues or take medication, there is a possibility of interaction so be sure to check with your doctor. Chaga is usually prepared as a tea or tincture. Tea can be made from freshly cut Chaga, but it is made more often from dried Chaga. It must be chopped into smaller pieces for drying unless the pieces are small. Drying at 110–125° is recommended. Dry it for at least twenty-four hours, then remove it for a few days so that any remaining interior moisture will stabilize. Then dry it again for another twenty-four hours or until it is bone dry. Then grind it with a meat grinder or gristmill. To make the powder even finer, use a heavy-duty blender.

Steeping ground or powdered Chaga in the normal way makes a pleasant tea. For the best medicinal benefit, there is evidence that decocting it by boiling for two or more hours is best. In either case, the tea is surprisingly good and has a more tealike flavor than mushroom flavor because of its tannic qualities.

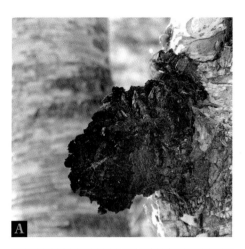

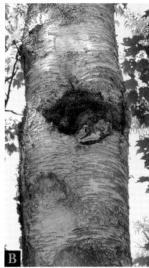

Figure A: A Chaga on white birch. **Figure B:** Sometimes specimens are too high to reach without a ladder. **Figure C:** An extra large Chaga on white birch. **Figure D:** This specimen is located right outside my house on a scarred birch. **Figure E:** A chopped-off specimen shows the yellow inner tissue.

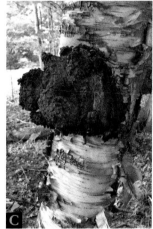

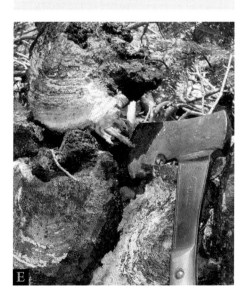

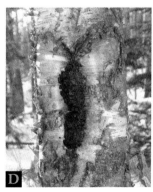

Chaga tea brews up darker than you would expect and blends very successfully with other teas and spices. As far as mushroom teas go, the flavor is excellent.

I have recently home brewed India pale ale, using Chaga as a replacement for boiling hops. It was exceptionally successful. About two heaping tablespoons of Chaga powder should be enough for a five-gallon wort. I decocted (long, hard boiling) the Chaga powder in a separate pot, adding it to the wort at the end. I was very pleased with its tannic qualities adding a positive note to the brew. Chaga ale's character was very different from the brew I made with the same recipe, substituting Reishi *(Ganoderma tsugae)* as the hop replacement. I will definitely make Chaga ale again soon.

A tincture of Chaga can be made using alcohol, such as eighty- to one-hundred-proof vodka, and water. To make the tincture: Fill up a container, such as a bottle or jar, at least one-third full with Chaga powder, then add vodka until it reaches the top of the container. Let the mixture sit for a few days or up to two weeks. Strain off the liquid and pour it through an unbleached coffee filter. When it has stopped dripping, squeeze the filter to yield a single extraction. You may take the leftover single-extracted Chaga mash (marc) and boil it (decoct) for one to two hours in water. Reduce the liquid by half and add it to your first extraction making a stronger double extraction maintaining an alcohol concentration of around twenty-five percent.

Comments: Chaga has been used as a tonic and tea by the Siberians for hundreds of years. Chaga contains inotodiol, betulin, and active polysaccharides that have various medicinal implications. A preparation called Befungin has been used in Russia for cancer treatment since the 1960s. I was surprised to see

Befungin being sold on eBay. The writer Aleksandr Solzhenitsyn believed it was Chaga that cured him of cancer in the 1950s.

Chaga can be used for dyeing textiles and paper and will yield a yellow or sepia color, depending on what mordant or modifier is used. *Inonotus obliquus* can also be used as tinder for fires and as incense. Dried Chaga burns well, but the incense is not particularly fragrant.

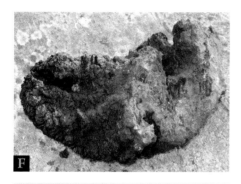

> ❧ **Figure F:** A dried specimen. ❧ **Figure G:** In winter, Chaga may have "snow hats" making the specimens easier to spot. ❧ **Figure H:** This Chaga is right next to the ground where excavating equipment scarred the tree.

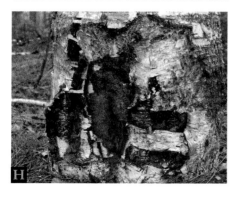

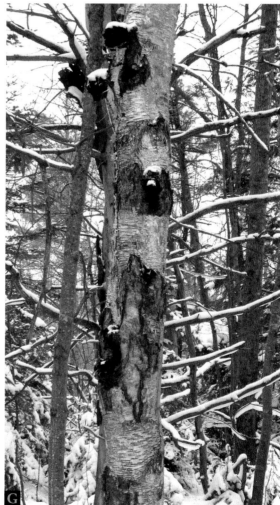

Section Six

Further Uses of Mushrooms

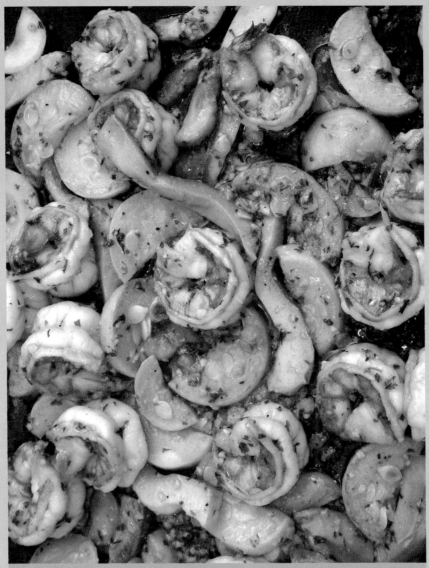

Freshwater shrimp with Chicken of the Woods, summer squash, garlic, oil, butter, and parsley.

Chapter Twenty-five

Preparing Mushrooms

Have you ever wondered what the mushroom field guides mean when they use a one-word description such as "choice," "good," or "edible" to rate a particular mushroom? I have often found myself wondering how this person cooked them. Were their mushrooms prepared alone, or mixed with other food products in a complex recipe?

I do not find it useful to know what a person may have thought of their Chanterelles in bouillabaisse or their Boletes in beef stew. I sometimes wonder if a rating of "slight bitterness" is the result of burned butter in the sauté pan. Recently, I tried *Hypholoma sublateritium,* the Brick Top for the first time. It was a "good" experience but mostly as a relatively neutral conveyance for butter. I have found that some mushrooms rated "edible" may have been picked at the wrong time, or they were cooked incorrectly. There are, though, many edible species that do fall into the "why bother" category. For instance, the Ash Tree Bolete *(Gyrodon meruloides)* smells and tastes like fresh tilled soil.

The edible species in this book are rated using four basic cooking processes. The basic processes detailed below are sautéing, tempura-frying, microwaving, and drying. By preparing the various species in these basic ways, you can learn how to use them best in more-complex recipes. Rather than offering recipes, the provided ratings and the comments on the species pages are meant to help guide your own culinary creativity. I have also included comments about other processes, such as grilling or boiling, on some of the species.

Like vegetables, mushrooms have different flavors and widely varying textures, colors, moisture content, and water absorbency. Hence, the various species respond to cooking processes differently. Many species only respond well to certain cooking techniques. Recipes in most cookbooks that call for some amount of mushrooms generally mean the White Button/Cremini/Portobello Mushrooms that have been offered in the grocery store for so many years. These are all-purpose mushrooms with an assertive mushroom flavor. Fortunately, though, more species of mushrooms are available today. However, because these other species may require different cooking techniques and/or may change the flavors of the finished dishes, they are not necessarily interchangeable in recipes.

If you have eaten many types of wild mushrooms, you might find recipes calling for half a pound of wild mushrooms about as sensible as an entry calling for half a pound of vegetables. Which ones? It would be more useful to think of wild mushrooms in a way you would think of fine wines. I believe many mushrooms can be associated with wines the way many recipes and foods are. A Chanterelle is ideal with a very subtle-flavored white wine, so it blends well with a chardonnay, Bordeaux, or Rhine. Similarly, a Chanterelle is best prepared in dishes you would associate with white wine, like chicken, fish, cheese, white sauces, and pasta. A Chanterelle would not work as well with steak or other red-wine types of foods. In comparison, the Porcini *(Boletus edulis),* a red-wine type of mushroom, has a strong woodsy flavor and is well suited in a stronger-flavored recipe, including steak, pork, venison, stew, gravy, and brown sauces. The stronger-flavored mushrooms have more versatility, but they may cancel out the flavor of the subtler-flavored species.

The following chart indicates which species work well with four types of wines.

Mushroom/Wine Compatibility

Species	Dry White Wine	German-style Wine	Sherry, Port, Marsala	Dry Red Wine
Chanterelle (*Cantharellus cibarius*)	Yes	Yes		
Black Trumpets (*Craterellus cornucopioides, C. cinereus,* and *C. foetidus*)	Yes	Yes	Yes	
Winter Chanterelle (*Craterellus tubaeformis*)	Yes	Yes		
Flame-colored Chanterelle (*Craterellus ignicolor*)	Yes	Yes		
Hedgehog Mushrooms (*Hydnum repandum* and *H. umbilicatum*)	Yes	Yes	Yes	
Horse Mushroom (*Agaricus arvensis*)			Yes	Yes
Meadow Mushroom (*Agaricus campestris*)			Yes	Yes
Parasol Mushroom (*Macrolepiota procera*)	Yes	Yes		
Shaggy Mane (*Coprinus comatus*)	Yes	Yes		
Matsutake (*Tricholoma magnivelare*)	Yes	Yes		

(chart continued on next page)

Species	Dry White Wine	German-style Wine	Sherry, Port, Marsala	Dry Red Wine
Blewit *(Lepista nuda)*	Yes	Yes		
Oyster Mushrooms *(Pleurotus ostreatus* and *P. populinus)*	Yes	Yes	Yes	
King Bolete *(Boletus edulis)*	Yes	Yes	Yes	Yes
Two-colored Bolete *(Boletus bicolor)*	Yes	Yes	Yes	
Boletus variipes (early-season *B. edulis* look-alike)	Yes	Yes	Yes	Yes
Painted Suillus *(Suillus pictus)*	Yes	Yes	Yes	
Chicken Fat Mushroom *(Suillus americanus)*	Yes	Yes	Yes	
Maitake *(Grifola frondosa)*	Yes	Yes	Yes	Yes
Chicken of the Woods *(Laetiporus sulphureus* and *L. cincinnatus)*	Yes	Yes	Yes	
Dryad's Saddle *(Polyporus squamosus)*	Yes	Yes		
Morels *(Morchella esculenta* and *M. elata)*	Yes	Yes	Yes	
Giant Puffball *(Calvatia gigantea)*				
Purple-spored Puffball *(Calvatia cyathiformis)*				
Lobster Mushroom *(Hypomyces lactifluorum)*	Yes	Yes	Yes	
Aborted Entoloma *(Entoloma abortivum)*	Yes	Yes	Yes	

I have seen well-known chefs on popular television shows do absolutely dreadful things with wild mushrooms. I have heard them say things that suggested they were not well versed in the mushrooms they were using. Do not bother with wild mushrooms if you are going to mix in White Button Mushrooms *(Agaricus bisporus)* from the store because they will overpower and make your wild mushrooms taste like the strong-flavored *Agaricus bisporus*. Many wild mushrooms are just too rare, subtle, and distinctive in flavor to be mixed or combined in certain ways. It makes as much sense as pouring Château Lafite-Rothschild Bordeaux into the holiday punch!

For safety's sake it is best to cook wild mushrooms thoroughly. There are plenty of bacteria in the outdoors that could make you sick, completely unrelated to the mushroom.

The Chanterelle *(Cantharellus cibarius)* is a truly wonderful mushroom when sautéed, but as tempura, the species may

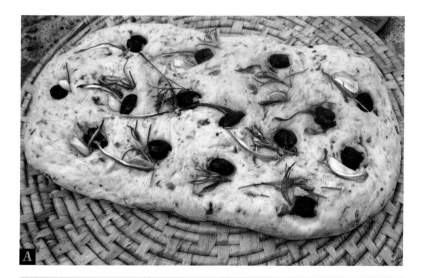

🍄 **Figure A:** Maitake/Hen of the Woods focaccia with Greek olives, red onions, garlic, and rosemary.

have less flavor and be a bit rubbery. As a dried product, *C. cibarius* does not reconstitute well for cooking but makes a truly fragrant, flavorful powder for seasoning when used in small quantity or flavoring when used in larger quantity. Chanterelle powder added to alfredo or other béchamel-based sauces is truly outstanding.

Oyster Mushrooms *(Pleurotus ostreatus* and *P. populinus)* are fairly tasty mushrooms when sautéed, though their flavor is a bit understated and their texture can be a bit chewy. When cooked with tempura batter, they are tender and flavorful. Oyster Mushrooms have a beautiful anise aroma when first picked. This aroma may dissipate somewhat within a few hours. If you can pick and cook them within a short time, the tempura will retain some of that anise character. The species is not very successful as a dried product. The texture is leathery when reconstituted; and as a powder, it is far less exciting than many other mushroom powders.

Maitake *(Grifola frondosa)* is one of the most versatile species. It responds well to sautéing, drying, and even microwaving. This species has a distinctive flavor that neither overpowers nor

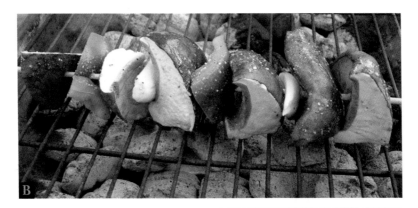

Figure B: *Boletus bicolor* shish kebab.

is overpowered. The Maitake has health and medicinal properties, as well. It is truly excellent.

King Boletes *(Boletus edulis)* are excellent sautéed but are truly wonderful dried and reconstituted. When powdered, they impart strong flavor. Among other uses, the powder is ideal for soup, gravy, meat loaf, and pasta sauce. However, it is easy to use too much.

Washing

Unless mushrooms are really clean and fresh, I am not of the "just brush 'em off" school. I do wash them. However, I do not float them in water because they can absorb unacceptable amounts of water that way. Sometimes a damp cloth is enough, but a sink sprayer can also work well especially if you do not spray the gills (if present) and you do not overdo it. I have tried compressed air with minor success. Compressed air can easily blow a hole in any delicate mushroom. The best way to clean a mushroom depends on the type. A lot of moisture in the sauté pan is not good. To avoid this, you can dry sauté any waterlogged mushrooms to drive off excess water by moving them about in a dry, hot pan for a while before adding oil or butter.

Often species in the *Agaricus* genus are so clean that they need no washing at all. *Agaricus campestris* is one of the most absorbent so you should wipe or wash them carefully. *A. arvensis* is not nearly as absorbent and may be washed more aggressively. I have always felt that we developed these attitudes about washing in part because of the *Agaricus bisporus* (White Button/Cremini/Portobello) we buy at the store that tend to absorb water and require careful washing.

For the past couple of years in Maine, we have had a plethora of slugs as a result of near record rainfall, mild winters, and other factors. Slugs often crawl across a cap overnight and eat a little bit. So I strongly recommend that you wipe, wash, and trim wherever necessary. If your mushrooms should take on some water, setting them on paper towels for a short while seems to help. The various species of mushrooms have different absorbency characteristics.

I have found quite a few older Chanterelles that were rained on quite a bit. That did not stop me.

Sautéing

Sautéing mushrooms can be tricky. All mushrooms tested are sautéed to the point where they are browned on the edges. Although some might prefer a "light" sauté, slight browning generally imparts richer flavor. Chanterelles, for example, create a yellow-orange juice in the pan. They should be sautéed until the juice is reduced and reclaimed.

Sautéing in butter is a favored technique. The amount of time and heat required to brown mushrooms, though, can cause the butter to burn, imparting a bitter flavor to the finished product.

It is better to sauté mushrooms until they are nearly finished in a neutral-flavored healthy oil, such as canola oil or olive oil. When they are almost done, add butter, which will slightly deglaze the pan and add extra flavor. Clarified butter can be used but it has a bit less flavor and will not deglaze the pan.

If you prefer using less oil, use a wok. Finishing the sauté with cream can be a simple but elegant approach to making a quick sauce. Once you understand the flavor characteristics of

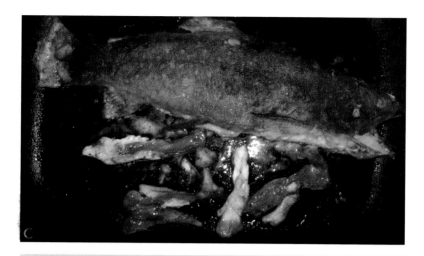

🍃 **Figure C:** Fresh native Maine brook trout with Chanterelles and Chicken of the Woods.

a particular mushroom, you may deglaze the pan with an appropriate wine as a finish. For example, last summer, I sautéed a particularly succulent Chicken of the Woods for a group of people and finished it with Riesling wine. Enjoyed by all, the Chicken of the Woods disappeared quite quickly. That day I was dubbed the Mushroom Maineiac.

If you find that you have too many mushrooms, duxelles is one solution. Duxelles is a paste used to flavor soups, sauces, and stuffing, or as a garnish. Escoffier's recipe for duxelles is made by sautéing finely chopping mushrooms or leftover stems and peelings in butter with onions and nutmeg, parsley, or other spices. Julia Child's recipe leaves out the onions. Consider using shallots, garlic, wine, or other spices. If some mushrooms need to have some moisture removed before cooking, wrap them in cloth and squeeze. Duxelles can then be frozen. Use ice trays or a muffin pan to freeze them into small blocks, then secure individually in plastic wrap for later use.

Tempura-Frying

Tempura is a light batter used for frying in oil. Oil temperature of 375° is best. I use a very basic recipe of flour, salt, and a pinch of baking powder or the prepackaged Japanese tempura from the supermarket. I use no milk (egg is optional), adding cold water and keeping the batter thin to yield a very crispy golden layer to the finished product.

Microwaving

Microwaving is a very neutral approach that uses no added ingredients and has advantages. Heating a meaty, medium- or large-sized mushroom in the microwave quite quickly renders it piping hot without driving out all the natural juice. I have microwaved Boletes, such as *Boletus bicolor,* and Blewits *(Lepista nuda)* very successfully. Be sure to point the stem upward so that any juice driven out is caught in the cap and watch the mushroom very closely. Depending on your microwave, a medium to large mushroom takes about 20 seconds or less.

Drying

Mushrooms are dried at 110–125° in either a dehydrator or gas oven. Often mushrooms do not fit well in a dehydrator unless you have an expensive Excalibur or similar large dehydrator. If you put too many in they often do not dry well. I find I can control my gas oven quite precisely by monitoring the temperature with a thermometer inside the oven.

I have a relatively simple General Electric gas stove. Although the lowest temperature on the oven knob is 200, I found I could achieve lower temperatures simply by setting it lower. Then I used an oven thermometer to determine the correct temperature setting and marked the knob for 110–120°.

I use flat pans with racks on top. Not only do I find it easier to dry unusual sizes and shapes of mushrooms in the oven, but I can also dry larger quantities. I acquired additional sliding racks so that I could really fill it to capacity. The oven also saves money by contributing to the heating of my house (I use propane for heat). Additionally, if you have fifty pounds of Maitake, you will need a gargantuan dehydrator.

Sun drying can also be tried with some species where weather permits. Black Trumpets, for example, dry quickly in hot sun, but a stiff wind could blow them away once they have dried. Air-drying works well with thinly sliced mushrooms using a needle and string to make a "mushroom necklace."

Dried mushrooms can be reconstituted, powdered, or even eaten dry in some cases. Use your favorite or texturally questionable dried mushrooms or leftover dried stems to make a very useful and flavorful powder: Chop bone-dry mushrooms in a blender or food processor, taking care not to breathe the dust that wafts out when you remove the cover. Powders impart a lot more flavor than dried whole mushrooms so do not use too much. Porcini/King Bolete powder, for instance, is very strong; and I once ruined a chicken dish by getting carried away.

Summary

This chart rates each cooking process on a scale from 1 to 100, with a score of 100 being the highest. These opinions are somewhat subjective, but many were shared by friends and relatives who "taste-tested" the species with me.

Cooking with Mushrooms

Species	Sauté	Tempura	Microwave	Dried
Chanterelle (*Cantharellus cibarius*)	95	75	60	90 (powdered)
Black Trumpets (*Craterellus cornucopioides, C. cinereus,* and *C. foetidus*)	99	95	X	97
Winter Chanterelle (*Craterellus tubaeformis*)	90	70	X	85 (powdered)
Flame-colored Chanterelle (*Craterellus ignicolor*)	90	70	X	85 (powdered)
Hedgehog Mushrooms (*Hydnum repandum* and *H. umbilicatum*)	92	90	90	90
Horse Mushroom (*Agaricus arvensis*)	94	95	85	90
Meadow Mushroom (*Agaricus campestris*)	90	92	80	90
Parasol Mushroom (*Macrolepiota procera*)	95	95	★	★
Shaggy Mane (*Coprinus comatus*)	92	92	★	★
Matsutake (*Tricholoma magnivelare*)	92	92	85	85
Blewit (*Lepista nuda*)	92	95	90	★
Oyster Mushrooms (*Pleurotus ostreatus* and *P. populinus*)	85	92	X	70 (powdered)

Species	Sauté	Tempura	Microwave	Dried
King Bolete (*Boletus edulis*)	92	85	90	95
Two-colored Bolete (*Boletus bicolor*)	93	90	90	90
Boletus variipes (early-season *B. edulis* look-alike)	85	80	★	★
Maitake (*Grifola frondosa*)	95	97	85	95
Chicken of the Woods (*Laetiporus sulphureus* and *L. cincinnatus*)	70–92 (variable)	90	75	★
Dryad's Saddle (*Polyporus squamosus*)	90 (when tender)	85	X	★
Morels (*Morchella esculenta* and *M. elata*)	95	95	★	95
Giant Puffball (*Calvatia gigantea*)	90	85	X	X
Purple-spored Puffball (*Calvatia cyathiformis*)	87	85	X	X
Lobster Mushroom (*Hypomyces lactifluorum*)	70–90 (variable)	80	★	80
Aborted Entoloma (*Entoloma abortivum*)	90	80	★	★

X indicates a process that should not be used
★ indicates a test not yet done

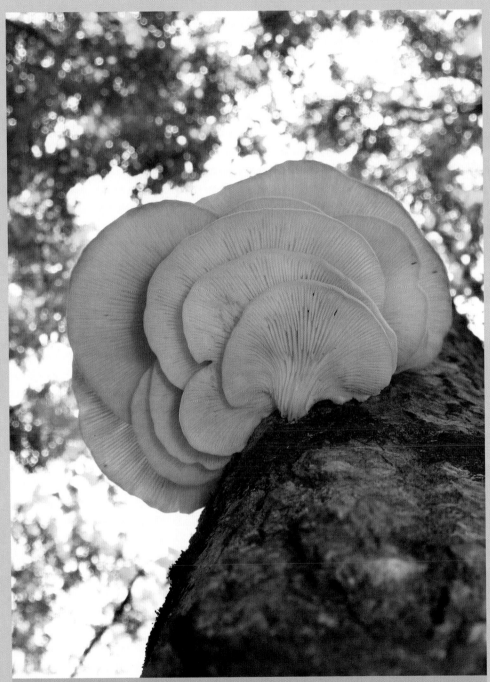

Oyster Mushrooms (*Pleurotus populinus*).

Chapter Twenty-six

Propagation Strategies

W hat do you do with the trimmings from your mushroom collecting? Do you throw your bottles away or do you recycle them? You would usually recycle them if you are being responsible. Well, you should do the same with your mushrooms.

After you bring home your mushrooms and find a few wormy caps, caps with bad spots, stem butts with bits of soil and mycelium attached, or mushrooms that are too old to eat, don't throw them away. Instead, take them outside and place them in similar habitats to where you found them. For example, I bury my Chanterelle stem butts and less than excellent caps under white pines and similar trees near my house and wormy Boletes under hemlocks or whatever type of trees and similar habitat I may have found them in. I do this with many species—except the Honey Mushroom, an aggressive parasite, that can destroy living trees.

It is true that a mushroom is just a fruit and that the mycelium usually continues to live when you pick the fruit body. However, by picking the specimen, you have removed the spores that the mushroom would have spread. Redistributing the trimmings may help to put some of the spores and mycelium back in the environment and create new areas of growth. Because I own a woodlot, I can do this easily; and I would certainly like to have these mushrooms growing around my house and supporting the health of my trees (as mycorrhizal species do) through symbiosis.

Slurries

Slurries are another way to distribute spores and tissue. Easy to make, slurries do not take much time and cost very little. To make a slurry that is loaded with millions of spores: Place mushroom caps in a container of water. Add a pinch of salt to inhibit bacterial growth. Let the mixture soak for twenty-four to forty-eight hours. After soaking, adding a small amount of molasses or sugar to the water will activate the spores within about twenty-four hours. Strain the mixture and pour the slurry where the mushrooms will have a chance to propagate. (You can also try putting mushroom caps in the blender with water to chop them finely for pouring.) I pour slurries onto stumps, wood chip beds, and other natural areas. I do not have a front lawn with grass. Mine is all wood chips. I am hoping my front yard will eventually support a variety of species. I also have snowmobile trails near my house, with a six-inch bed of wood-chips on them as well as areas with tons of mixed wood and dirt biomass that I have applied slurries to.

Spore Prints

Making a spore print is often an essential part of identifying the species. Spore prints are usually made on glass or paper; however, a white spore print on white paper is not useful. I like to make my spore prints on microscope slides. Simply place the cap onto the glass or paper and wait for spores to fall—usu-ally many will fall within a few hours. Placing a glass or bowl over the mushroom and slide will prevent too much spore dispersal and may give a better spore print. I then place a clean slide on top and tape them together with Magic Tape, which is easy to write on and to remove.

Spore prints can be used to make slurries or cultures. Because local wild species are well adapted to the weather and ecology, it is wise to try to propagate from local specimens only instead of spores or cultures from other parts of the country or world. Cultures can be made fairly easily at home in petri dishes with sterile agar as a growing medium, both of which are available on eBay for a reasonable price. Creating cultures is not that difficult if you take steps to be clean. You can make or buy a tabletop inoculation chamber quite inexpensively.

Plug Spawn

Plug spawn is used for inoculating logs or similar substances with mushroom mycelium. Plug spawn is usually made with fluted birch dowels used for joining the components of fine wood furniture. Mushroom mycelium from a culture or other form of spawn is introduced into clean or sterile saturated dowel plugs. After the mycelium completely colonizes the plugs, they are ready to use for inoculating clean usually hardwood logs. Holes are drilled in the logs and the plugs are hammered in and optionally sealed over with bee's wax.

Sometimes I have successfully used nonsterile materials. For instance, I have taken the caps of Oyster Mushrooms and placed them over a canning jar filled with water-soaked wooden dowel plugs, which produced vigorous growth from the spore fall. I have placed the stem butts of wild, freshly picked Oyster Mushrooms in a jar of water-soaked dowel plugs. After the plugs are fully colonized, I hammer the dowel plugs into holes drilled into logs, resulting in outstanding growth of mushrooms. I keep a few dozen logs in a shady area outside my house and enjoy fresh Shiitake and Oyster Mushrooms during the warmer months with my family. I have also grown Shiitake on unsterilized hardwood sawdust from a local wood harvester. I have experienced a number of failures but it can be done.

Transplantation

Digging up a specimen with the soil and mycelium intact is another way to transplant mushrooms. The soil contains beneficial bacteria and other elements necessary for the specimen's growth. To preserve the integrity of the soil ball, dig up your mushroom with a garden trowel and place it in a small flowerpot or bag until you can transplant the mushroom to the desired place. When you are ready to transplant to another suitable locations, use a shovel to pick up a mycelial mass to plant it in wood chips or compost or soft soil. An environment similar to the one the mushroom came from is best. Transplantation may only work occasionally.

Other Growth Strategies

I often collect old or wormy specimens that I would like to grow on my property. I have thrown a lot of overripe Puffballs and other species out toward my leech field and other areas. I have also placed old Oyster Mushrooms, Chicken of the Woods, Maitake, and Dryad's Saddle onto the recently cut stumps that were created when I had some selective cutting done on my woodlot. I had this done not only to improve the health of the woods but also with an eye toward further myco-logical experimentation. The trees that were cut were sold for firewood, pulp, biomass, and lumber. I kept most of the extra large trees and dead or dying "woodpecker trees." Fortunately, this selective-cutting process was a success. Additionally, the wood I had removed for stump inoculation improved the over-story by allowing a greater amount of light to reach the more-valuable conifers, birches, oak, ash, and other more unusual hardwood trees.

I have purchased chainsaw oil, with spores mixed into canola oil, from Fungi Perfecti to use as bar and chain oil. Not only do you always broadcast spores this way, canola oil is much more environmentally friendly. Currently, millions of gallons of petroleum chainsaw oil pollute the environment each year. Further, petroleum-based oils can cause health problems, including cancer as well as respiratory and skin problems. I have made my own oil with spores from a variety of species, such as Oyster Mushrooms, local to my area. Two or three large Oyster Mushrooms left on a sheet of glass will produce a phenomenal number of spores, which may easily drop sev-eral grams that should be literally billions of spores. In theory this amount should be enough for gallons of oil and hundreds of other applications.

Chapter Twenty-seven

Dyeing with Mushrooms

A s you have read, numerous species of mushrooms can be used to dye wool, some fabrics, and other fibers. Paper can be made from some species and mushroom papers can then be dyed with other mushrooms for a unique, textured, colored paper suitable for art applications.

At the 2007 Northeast Mycological Annual Samuel Ristich Foray in Orono, Maine, I saw a truly impressive display of dyed wool made by Anne Williams of Stonington, Maine. For years, she has been experimenting using mushrooms as dyes, and the results of her efforts are truly excellent. Using numerous mushrooms that no one else has and dozens of species, Anne has created many beautiful, different-colored wools.

As the following chart indicates, simple natural mordants/modifiers—such as salt water, vinegar, ammonia, a copper pot, and a rusty iron pot—are used. For four to five ounces of wool, up to half of a plastic shopping bag of mushrooms is generally required. About twelve ounces or more of mushrooms per four ounces of wool is a good way to measure (3:1). An alkaline solution is best in most cases. When using ammonia, about one cup per four ounces of wool should be used (2:1). Dye-maker's Polypore *(Phaeolus schweinitzii)* and Lobster Mushrooms *(Hypomyces lactifluorum)* can be used in smaller quantities.

Dyes can be made from mushrooms you find that are not edible, slightly gone by, or wormy. This can add a new dimension to your collecting.

Below is a chart of mushroom species, mordants/modifiers, and the resulting colors of Anne Williams's dyed wool.

Dyeing Wool with Mushrooms

Species	Mordant/Modifier	Color Produced
Chanterelle (*Cantharellus cibarius*)	ammonia	muted yellow
Flame-colored Chanterelle (*Craterellus ignicolor*)	ammonia	muted yellow
Horse Mushroom (*Agaricus arvensis*)	salt water iron pot	yellow-tan gray-green
Meadow Mushroom (*Agaricus campestris*)	salt water iron pot	yellow-tan gray-green
Shaggy Mane (*Coprinus comatus*)	iron pot ammonia	bayberry gray-green
Blewit (*Lepista nuda*)	ammonia/copper pot	grass-green
Oyster Mushroom (*Pleurotus ostreatus*)	ammonia/iron pot	gray-green
King Bolete (*Boletus edulis*)	ammonia	chrome-mustard
Maitake (*Grifola frondosa*)	ammonia	soft yellow
Chicken of the Woods (*Laetiporus sulphureus* and *L. cincinnatus*)	ammonia	orange
Giant Puffball (*Calvatia gigantea*)	ammonia	red-brown

Species	Mordant/Modifier	Color Produced
Purple-spored Puffball (*Calvatia cyathiformis*)	ammonia	rust red
Orange-staining Puffball (*Calvatia ruboflava*)	vinegar	rust red
Lobster Mushroom (*Hypomyces lactifluorum*)	ammonia	cinnamon pink to red
Reishi (*Ganoderma tsugae*)	ammonia	rust
Artist's Conk (*Ganoderma applanatum*)	ammonia	rust
Turkey Tail (*Trametes versicolor*)	ammonia	brown
Dye-maker's Polypore (*Phaeolus schweinitzii*)	ammonia ammonia/copper pot ammonia/iron pot salt water	orange deep green red rust brilliant yellow
Reddening Lepiota (*Lepiota americana*)	salt water ammonia	pink beige deeper tones

References

Books

Arora, David. *Mushrooms Demystified: A Comprehensive Guide to the Fleshy Fungi.* 2nd ed. Berkeley: Ten Speed Press, 1986.

Barron, George. *Mushrooms of Northeast North America: Midwest to New England.* Edmonton, Canada: Lone Pine Publishing, 1999.

Bessette, Alan E., Arleen Rainis Bessette, and David W. Fischer. *Mushrooms of Northeastern North America.* Syracuse, NY: Syracuse University Press, 1997.

Bessette, Alan E., William C. Roody, and Arleen Rainis Bessette. *North American Boletes: A Color Guide to the Fleshy Pored Mushrooms.* Syracuse, NY: Syracuse University Press, 2000.

Fergus, Charles L. *Common Edible and Poisonous Mushrooms of the Northeast.* Mechanicsburg, PA: Stackpole Books, 2003.

Hobbs, Christopher. *Medicinal Mushrooms: An Exploration of Tradition, Healing, and Culture.* Santa Cruz, CA: Botanica Press, 1995.

Kuo, Michael. *Morels.* Ann Arbor: University of Michigan Press, 2005.

Lincoff, Gary H. *National Audubon Society Field Guide to North American Mushrooms.* New York: Alfred A. Knopf, 1981.

Miller, Orson K., and Hope Miller. *North American Mushrooms: A Field Guide to Edible and Inedible Fungi.* Guilford, CT: Falcon Guide, 2006.

Phillips, Roger. *Mushrooms and Other Fungi of North America.* Buffalo, NY: Firefly Books, 2005.

Preuss, Harry G., and Sensuke Konno. *Maitake Magic.* Topanga, CA: Freedom Press, 2002.

Russell, Bill. *Field Guide to the Wild Mushrooms of Pennsylvania and the Mid-Atlantic.* University Park: Pennsylvania State University Press, 2006.

Stamets, Paul. *Growing Gourmet and Medicinal Mushrooms.* 3rd ed. Berkeley: Ten Speed Press, 2000.

———. *Mycelium Running: How Mushrooms Can Help Save the World.* Berkeley: Ten Speed Press, 2005.

Medical studies

Asai, Y., K. Takaori, T. Yamamoto, and T. Ogawa. 2005. Protein-bound polysaccharide isolated from basidiomycetes inhibits endotoxin-induced activation by blocking lipopolysaccharide-binding protein and CD14 functions. *FEMS Immunology and Medical Microbiology* 2005 Jan 1;43(1):91 8. Department of Oral Microbiology, Asahi University School of Dentistry, 1851-1 Hozumi, Mizuho, Gifu 501-0296, Japan.

Gu, Y. H., and G. Sivam. 2006. Cytotoxic effect of oyster mushroom *Pleurotus ostreatus* on human androgen-independent prostate cancer PC-3 cells. *Journal of Medicinal Food* 2006 Summer;9(2):196–204. School of Natural Health Sciences, Bastyr University, Kenmore, Washington, USA. yuhuang@bastyr.edu.

Ho, C. Y., C. F. Kim, K. N. Leung, K. P. Fung, T. F. Tse, H. Chan, and C. B. Lau. 2005. Differential anti-tumor activity of *Coriolus versicolor* (Yunzhi) extract through p53 and/or Bcl-2-dependent apoptotic pathway in human breast cancer cells. *Journal of Cancer Biology and Therapy* 2005 Jun;4(6):638–44. Epub 2005 Jun 8. School of Pharmacy, The Chinese University of Hong Kong, Shatin, New Territories, Hong Kong.

Ho, C. Y., C. F. Kim, K. N. Leung, K. P. Fung, T. F. Tse, H. Chan, and C. B. Lau. 2006. *Coriolus versicolor* (Yunzhi) extract attenuates growth of human leukemia xenografts and induces apoptosis through the mitochondrial pathway. *Oncology Reports* 2006

Sep;16(3):609–16. School of Pharmacy, The Chinese University of Hong Kong, Hong Kong, PR China.

Kim, Y. O., H. W. Park, J. H. Kim, J. Y. Lee, S. H. Moon, and C. S. Shin. 2006. Anti-cancer effect and structural characterization of endo-polysaccharide from cultivated mycelia of *Inonotus obliquus*. *Life Sciences* 2006 May 30;79(1):72–80. Epub 2006 Feb 3. Department of Biotechnology, College of Engineering, Yonsei University, Shinchon-dong, Seodaemoon-gu, Seoul 120-749, South Korea.

Kobayashi, H., K. Matsunaga, and Y. Oguchi. Antimetastatic effects of PSK (Krestin), a protein-bound polysaccharide obtained from basidiomycetes: an overview. *Cancer Epidemiology Biomarkers & Prevention,* Vol 4, Issue 3 275–281, Copyright © 1995 by American Association for Cancer Research. Health Science University of Hokkaido, Japan.

Kodama, N., K. Komuta, N. Sakai, and H. Namba. 2002. Effects of D-Fraction, a polysaccharide from *Grifola frondosa* on tumor growth involve activation of NK cells. *Biological & Pharmaceutical Bulletin* 2002 Dec;25(12):1647–50. Department of Microbial Chemistry, Kobe Pharmaceutical University, Japan. n-kokama@kobepharma-u.ac.jp.

Lavi, I., D. Friesem, S. Geresh, Y. Hadar, and B. Schwartz. 2006. An aqueous polysaccharide extract from the edible mushroom *Pleurotus ostreatus* induces anti-proliferative and pro-apoptotic effects on HT-29 colon cancer cells. *Cancer Letters* 2006 Nov 28;244(1):61–70. Epub 2006 Jan 18. Institute of Biochemistry, Food Science and Nutrition, Faculty of Agricultural, Food and Environmental Quality Sciences, The Hebrew University of Jerusalem, P.O. Box 12, Rehovot 76100, Israel.

Moradali, M. F., H. Mostafavi, G. A. Hejaroude, A. S. Tehrani, M. Abbasi, and S. Ghods. 2006. Investigation of potential antibacterial properties of methanol extracts from fungus *Ganoderma applanatum. Chemotherapy* 2006;52(5):241–4. Epub 2006 Aug 4. Plant Protection Department, Faculty of Agriculture, Tehran University, Karaj, Iran.

Peng, Y., and L. Zhang. 2003. Characterization of a polysaccharide-protein complex from *Ganoderma tsugae* mycelium by size-exclusion chromatography combined with laser light scattering. *Journal of Biochemical and Biophysical Methods* 2003 Jun 30;56(1–3):243–52. Department of Chemistry, Wuhan University, Wuhan 430072, China.

Sarangi, I., D. Ghosh, S. K. Bhutia, S. K. Mallick, and T. K. Maiti. 2006. Anti-tumor and immunomodulating effects of *Pleurotus ostreatus* mycelia-derived proteoglycans. *International Immunopharmacology* 2006 Aug;6(8):1287–97. Epub 2006 May 9. Department of Biotechnology, Indian Institute of Technology, Kharagpur 721302, West Bengal, India.

Shim, S. H., J. Ryu, J.S. Kim, S. S. Kang, Y. Xu, S. H. Jung, Y. S. Lee, S. Lee, and K. H. Shin. 2004. New lanostane-type triterpenoids from *Ganoderma applanatum. Journal of Natural Products* 2004 Jul;67(7):1110–3. Natural Products Research Institute and College of Pharmacy, Seoul National University, 28 Yeun-gun-dong, Chongno-gu, Seoul 110-460, Korea.

Talpur, N., B. Echard, A. Dadgar, S. Aggarwal, C. Zhuang, D. Bagchi, and H. G. Preuss. 2002. Effects of Maitake mushroom fractions on blood pressure of Zucker fatty rats. *Research Communications in Molecular Pathology & Pharmacology* 2002;112 (1–4):68–82. Department of Physiology, Medicine and Pathology, Georgetown University Medical Center, Washington, DC 20057.

Talpur, N. A., B. W. Echard, A. Y. Fan, O. Jaffari, D. Bagchi, and H. G. Preuss. 2002. Antihypertensive and metabolic effects of whole Maitake mushroom powder and its fractions in two rat strains. *Molecular and Cellular Biochemistry* 2002 Aug;237 (1–2):129–36.

Department of Physiology and Biophysics, Georgetown University Medical Center, Washington, DC 20007.

Yue, G. G., K. P. Fung, G. M. Tse, P. C. Leung, and C. B. Lau. 2006. Comparative studies of various *Ganoderma* species and their different parts with regard to their antitumor and immunomodulating activities in vitro. *Journal of Alternative and Complementary Medicine* 2006 Oct;12(8):777–89. Institute of Chinese Medicine, The Chinese University of Hong Kong, Shatin, Hong Kong, China.

Index

About the Author

A former commercial photographer, David Spahr has collected, photographed, and eaten wild mushrooms for thirty-five years and is a member of the Maine Mycological Association. He maintains a Web site devoted to the subject, www.mushroom collecting.com, and also moderates the discussion group at http://groups.yahoo.com/group/NortheastMushrooms/. Spahr graduated from Hartwick College in 1973 with a degree in art and has continued his studies at the University of Maine. In addition to his mushroom-related pursuits, Spahr holds a second degree black belt in Tae Kwon Do and has been a practitioner and teacher of Tai Chi for twenty-six years.